Water Fun

Terri Lees

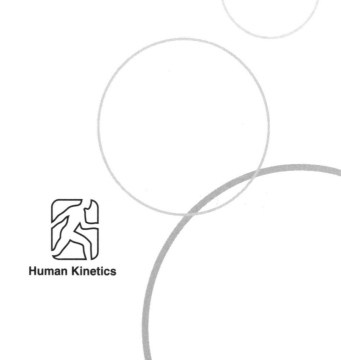

Human Kinetics

Library of Congress Cataloging-in-Publication Data

Lees, Terri.
  Water fun / Terri Lees.
    p. cm.
  Rev. ed. of: Water fun and fitness. c1995.
  ISBN-13: 978-0-7360-6378-4 (soft cover)
  ISBN-10: 0-7360-6378-1 (soft cover)
  1. Aquatic exercises. 2. Aquatic exercises--Health aspects. 3. Aquatic sports--Safety measures. I. Lees, Terri. Water fun and fitness. II. Title.
  GV838.53.E94E44 2007
  613.7'16--dc22   2006032666

ISBN-10: 0-7360-6378-1
ISBN-13: 978-0-7360-6378-4

This book is a revised edition of *Water Fun and Fitness,* published in 1995 by Human Kinetics, Inc.

The Web addresses cited in this text were current as of October 2006, unless otherwise noted.

Acquisitions Editor: Patricia Sammann; **Managing Editor:** Kathleen Bernard; **Assistant Editor:** Heather M. Tanner; **Copyeditor:** Jacqueline Eaton Blakley; **Proofreader:** Bethany J. Bentley; **Permission Manager:** Carly Breeding; **Graphic Designer:** Nancy Rasmus; **Graphic Artist:** Yvonne Griffith; **Cover Designer:** Keith Blomberg; **Photographer (cover):** Neil S. Bernstein and Terri Lees (corner photo); **Art Manager:** Kelly Hendren; **Illustrator:** Bruce Morton; **Printer:** United Graphics

Human Kinetics books are available at special discounts for bulk purchase. Special editions or book excerpts can also be created to specification. For details, contact the Special Sales Manager at Human Kinetics.

Printed in the United States of America   10 9 8 7 6 5 4 3 2 1

Human Kinetics
Web site: www.HumanKinetics.com

United States: Human Kinetics
P.O. Box 5076
Champaign, IL 61825-5076
800-747-4457
e-mail: humank@hkusa.com

Canada: Human Kinetics
475 Devonshire Road Unit 100
Windsor, ON N8Y 2L5
800-465-7301 (in Canada only)
e-mail: orders@hkcanada.com

Europe: Human Kinetics
107 Bradford Road, Stanningley
Leeds LS28 6AT, United Kingdom
+44 (0) 113 255 5665
e-mail: hk@hkeurope.com

Australia: Human Kinetics
57A Price Avenue
Lower Mitcham, South Australia 5062
08 8372 0999
e-mail: liaw@hkaustralia.com

New Zealand: Human Kinetics
Division of Sports Distributors NZ Ltd.
P.O. Box 300 226 Albany
North Shore City
Auckland
0064 9 448 1207
e-mail: info@humankinetics.co.nz

To my husband who loves me just as I am;

to my children and grandchildren who are always okay with me being a "dork";

to all of the wonderful people who played along and provided valuable feedback;

to all of the teachers, coaches, and "AquaNutz" who jumped, feet first, into the waves; and

to all of the people who will continue the ripple effect of water fun and fitness.

May the joy of participation bless you for many years to come.

contents

activity finder

The Fitness Activity Finder is organized so that you can take a quick look and easily identify the activities in chapters 4 and 5 that will help you reach your fitness goals.

Fitness Activity Finder

Activity Type

AW = Arm works

AB = Aqua basics

SA = Sport aqua

PSS = Partner stunts and skills

RG = Relay game

TG = Tag game

IE = Individual event

TE = Team event

Fitness Focus

WU = Warm-up or cool-down

CE = Cardiorespiratory endurance

IT = Interval training

ME = Muscular endurance

Fitness Activity Finder

Name	Activity type	Fitness focus	Equipment	Variations	Page
Balloon Relay	RG	IT	Yes	Yes	88
Beach Ball Volleyball	TE	CE	Yes	Yes	100
Butterfly	AW	ME	No	No	36
Butt Kicker	AB	WU	No	No	46
Chest Pass	SA	ME	Yes	Yes	57
Cross-Country Ski	AB	ME, CE	No	Yes	46
Curl	AW	ME	No	Yes	36
Defensive Slide	SA	ME, CE	No	Yes	52
Figure Eight (Sculling)	AW	ME	No	No	40
Fill the Hole	IE	WU	No	Yes	100
Flag Tag	TG	ME, IT	Yes	Yes	91
Follow the Leader	IE	WU, ME, CE, IT	No	Yes	94
Front Kick	SA	ME	No	No	65
Fusion Tag	TG	IT	No	Yes	92
Grapevine	SA	ME, CE	No	No	53
Hill Topper	SA	ME, CE, IT	No	No	54
Hydro-Triathlon	IE	ME, CE, IT	No	Yes	105
Jumping Jack	AB	ME, WU	No	Yes	47
Jump and Spin	PSS, IE	IT	No	Yes	76
Kickboard Cruising	IE	ME	Yes	Yes	78
Kickboard Rowing	AW	ME	Yes	No	40
Kicker	AB	ME, CE	No	Yes	44
Lateral Raise	AW	ME	No	Yes	39
Marching and Jogging	AB	ME, CE, IT	No	Yes	43
Medley Dash Relay	RG	IT	No	Yes	86
Mountain Climber	AB	ME, CE	No	No	44
Musical Noodles or Kickboards	IE	CE	Yes	Yes	98

(continued)

(continued)

Name	Activity type	Fitness focus	Equipment	Variations	Page
Noodle Bicycle	IE	ME, CE, IT	Yes	No	83
Noodle Locomotion	IE	CE, IT	Yes	Yes	80
Object Retrieval Race	TE	IT	Yes	Yes	95
Partner Jump Turn	PSS	IT	No	No	78
Partner Locomotion	PSS	CE, IT	No	Yes	75
Partner Relay	RG	IT	No	No	86
Pigeon Race	IE	IT	No	Yes	97
Pinball Tag	TG	IT	No	Yes	93
Pool Push-Up	AW	ME	No	No	37
Power Jog	SA	ME, CE, IT	No	Yes	50
Power Knee Lift	SA	ME, CE, IT	No	Yes	55
Pull-Down	AW	ME	No	Yes	38
Punches	SA	ME	No	No	62
Push Me, Pull You	PSS	ME, IT	Yes	Yes	85
Rebound	SA	ME, IT	No	Yes	59
Rickshaw Relay	RG	IT	Yes	Yes	89
Rope Jump	SA	ME, CE	No	Yes	56
Scissors	AB	ME, CE	No	Yes	45
Side Kick	SA	ME	No	No	65
Ski Jump	SA	ME	No	No	61
Skip Bounding	SA	ME, IT	No	No	57
Sock and Shirt Relay	RG	IT	Yes	Yes	87
Survivor Challenge	TE	IT	Yes	Yes	102
Swim Strokes	AW	ME	No	Yes	35
Tandem Bicycle	PSS	ME, CE, IT	Yes	Yes	83
Tandem Noodle Jacks	PSS	ME	Yes	Yes	84
Tandem Noodle Ski	PSS	ME, CE, IT	Yes	Yes	82
Tarzan Swim	IE	ME	Yes	No	81

Name	Activity type	Fitness focus	Equipment	Variations	Page
Three-Person Weave	SA	ME, CE	Yes	Yes	58
Three-Step Jump Stop	SA	ME, CE	No	Yes	51
Tire Run	SA	ME, CE	No	No	53
Tug-of-War	TE	IT	Yes	Yes	99
Wave Gauntlet	IE, TE	ME, IT	Yes	Yes	103
Whistle Stop Stunt Race	IE	IT	No	Yes	101

With the Swim Activity Finder, you can choose those water adjustment activities, stunts and skills, swimming games, and fitness swimming formats that work best for the swimming abilities of your class.

Swim Activity Finder

Activity Type

WA = Water adjustment or warm-up

ST = Stunts and skills

SG = Swimming games

FS = Fitness swimming

Prerequisites

L = Independent locomotion

S = Submersion (includes breath control and eyes opened underwater)

F = Unsupported floating or gliding on front or back

SC = Sculling

SW = Swimming

Swim Activity Finder

Name	Activity type	Prerequisites	Equipment	Variations	Page
Aqua Man Relay	SG	L, S	No	No	151
Ball Relay	SG	SW	Yes	Yes	156
Baseball	SG	L, SW	Yes	Yes	151
Big Splash Contest	SG	L, S, SW	Yes	Yes	161
Blowing a Floating Object	WA	L	Yes	Yes	115
Burn Out	ST	S, SW	No	Yes	127
Catch-Up Swim	FS	SW	No	Yes	163
Chain Dolphin	ST	S, SW, SC	No	No	147
Circles Around the Pool	FS	SW	No	Yes	165
Circles in the Lane	FS	SW	No	No	165
Corkscrew	ST	S, SW	No	Yes	134
Crack the Whip	WA	S, L	No	Yes	124
Deep-Water Gymnastics	ST	S, SW, SC	No	No	144
Down the River	ST	L, F, SC	No	No	137
Fin Tag	SG	S, SW	Yes	No	154
Fire Pole	WA	S	Yes	Yes	122
Fish Flop	WA	L	No	No	119
Flip-Flops	ST	L	Yes	Yes	129
Float Patterns	ST	L, F, SC	No	Yes	139
Follow the Leader	SG	F, SW, SC	No	Yes	149
Four Corners	FS	SW	No	Yes	164
Human Cork	WA	S	No	No	118
Hydrojets	ST	L, F	No	No	128
Independent Kicking	ST	L	Yes	Yes	125
Kicking War	ST	S, F	No	Yes	132
Leapfrog	ST	L, S	No	Yes	144
Life Jacket Water Polo	SG	SW	Yes	Yes	158

Name	Activity type	Prerequisites	Equipment	Variations	Page
Listening Underwater	WA	S	Yes	No	116
Log Roll	ST	S, F	No	No	131
Lying on the Bottom	WA	S	No	No	121
Medley Relay	SG	SW	No	Yes	155
Mini-Triathlon/ Biathlon	FS	SW	No	Yes	167
Object Retrieval	WA	L, S	Yes	Yes	123
Partner Handstands	ST	L, S	No	No	143
Planking	ST	S, F, SC	No	No	140
Porpoise Dives	ST	L, S	No	No	130
Rag Tag	SG	L, S, SW	Yes	Yes	152
Sculling	ST	F	No	Yes	134
Sitting on the Bottom	WA	S	No	No	121
Sky Ball	WA	L	Yes	Yes	117
Splash the Teacher	WA	L	No	No	116
Squid Swim	ST	L, S	No	No	131
Stuff It	ST	L	Yes	No	140
Swim Across the English Channel	FS	SW	No	Yes	166
Swim the Waves	SG	S, SW	Yes	Yes	157
Tandem Relay	SG	SW	No	No	157
Tandem Swim	ST	SW, SC	No	Yes	138
Teeter-Totter	WA	L, S	No	No	120
Thread the Needle	ST	L, S	No	No	133
Underwater Hockey	SG	L, S, SW	Yes	Yes	160
Water Barrel	WA	L	No	No	118
Water Gymnastics	ST	L, S	No	Yes	141
Wheelbarrow	ST	L, S	No	Yes	126
Whistle Stop Stunt Race	SG	S, SW, SC	No	Yes	150
Zigzag Swim	FS	SW	No	Yes	164

preface

The first edition of this book, *Water Fun and Fitness,* was written to address the needs of aquatic specialists, recreation professionals, youth agency personnel, and school physical educators working with large groups with varied swimming abilities. At that time, ideas for learn-to-swim activities for these groups were scarce, so the book focused on teaching fun lead-up skills to help children learn to swim. Although fun lead-up skills to swimming are still important in this new edition, the focus has shifted to water exercises for people of all ages, exercises that will use available pool space efficiently and will help address the ever-increasing obesity crisis.

Adults, even athletes, have discovered the benefits of water exercise, finding new freedom, friendships, and fitness alternatives in the water. Besides being a lifelong way to stay fit, water exercise can also help participants learn to swim and be safe in the water. Water exercise is a fun, challenging, and rewarding way to achieve these goals.

This second edition emphasizes games and activities that keep fitness fun. The book has been expanded to include more basic water exercises performed in a vertical position and more workout options that don't require participants to fully submerge themselves in the water. It still has the same reader-friendly collection of stunts, skills, and games that can make learning to swim safe, exciting, and fun. And it also includes the same basic water adjustment and stroke readiness skills needed to help participants make the transition from water exercise to swimming.

Chapter 1 introduces the benefits of water fitness and describes why water works so well as a fitness medium. It also includes an overview of the special qualities of the water and explains how each can help one improve and maintain fitness while having fun and learning to swim.

Next come the fitness basics. In chapter 2 we learn the elements of a water workout. It includes an easy-to-follow readiness test to make sure one is able to participate safely in the water using basic locomotor skills, and it provides guidelines for cardiorespiratory and muscular endurance training using aqua basic exercise and interval formats. At the end of the chapter is a section on how to adapt the basics and games activities that will follow to meet group and individual needs.

In chapter 3 the emphasis is on aquatic program safety. It includes a facility safety checklist, a discussion of appropriate rules and regulations for a safe program, and personal safety information for both instructors and participants. The reader is encouraged to teach the basic water safety skills to increase participant awareness and promote safe play and skill learning.

Basic water activities in chapter 4 cover arm movements, traveling options, and sport aqua ideas. This chapter also outlines how to design a fun and challenging water fitness workout using those activities. We have included several workout formats to make it easier to apply the principles outlined in this chapter.

The aqua basics are turned into "funderful" game activities in chapter 5, beginning with ideas for individual stunts and partner activities that can be incorporated into various relays, tags, and large-group games. All of the activities in this chapter are for vertical play with the face out of the water, but some include options for those who can swim.

Teaching participants to swim is the goal in the final chapter, helping them to make a successful transition from exercise in the vertical position to swimming in the horizontal position. To help the instructor and the swimmers, the chapter includes a simple readiness test. Readers are encouraged to spend time teaching participants the basic personal safety skills so participants can be comfortable and safe as they learn to swim and have fun playing the swimming games that conclude the chapter. The activities should be challenging and fun for both old and new swimmers and should teach all participants safety skills they can use for a lifetime.

Appendixes at the end of the book provide the reader with additional aids. There's a descriptive list of aquatic equipment, along with a list of equipment sources. There's also a list of associations related to water exercise and safety, as well as a sheet for checking preswimming skills.

Most of the activities presented in this book are conducted in shallow water and require very little (or no) swimming skill. However, the deep-water variations and partner stunts and skills will be novel and challenging for swimmers. Many of these activities have been used with developmentally disabled youth and adults, and most have been tried in older-adult aquatic fitness classes in community recreation. Those who conduct the activities in *Water Fun* don't have to have exceptional swimming skills. They only need to care about giving participants a safe aquatic learning experience so that participants become comfortable enough in the water to learn fitness and swimming skills and have *waves* of fun doing it.

chapter 1

Introduction to Water Fitness and Swimming

The water is an exciting, fresh medium for activity. It has a natural beauty that lures people of all ages into participation. In this chapter you will discover some of the reasons why water works and why exercise in the water is one of the fastest-growing fitness activities. You'll find that a games approach to water workouts will improve participation and enhance fitness, and you'll recognize that water fun and fitness activities can prepare even apprehensive beginners for a more comfortable learn-to-swim experience. Your participants will be so comfortable and so supported by the water that they'll try beginning swimming skills without ever realizing that they are learning. And through all of the fun, you will be encouraging and supporting the development of a fitness habit that will last a lifetime.

Why Water Works

Water has unique qualities that make it a near-perfect workout environment. *Buoyancy* (the upward lift of the water) gives one a feeling of weightlessness and takes pressure off the joints so that even someone who has an injury or disability can enjoy physical activity without increased joint pain. Buoyancy supports you, assists movement toward the surface (knee lifts and jogging are made easier), and creates resistance when you pull body parts toward the bottom of the pool (as in returning to the start position of a jumping jack).

Buoyancy combines with *hydrostatic pressure* to assist with standing balance. This allows people with balance and coordination difficulties to participate actively without the fear of falling. Hydrostatic pressure is exerted on the body from all sides. It is responsible for the initial pressure you feel on your chest and the resistance to breathing you experience when you first enter the water. It helps keep blood from collecting in the feet and ankles and helps massage the tissues as you move in the water.

Water also has weight and density that create *multidimensional resistance*, meaning that you will feel the heaviness of the water in every direction you move. The resistance of the water slows movement and makes exercise safer, and at the same time requires more effort than land-based exercise at the same speed. A unique feature of water resistance is that it can be increased or decreased (manipulated) at will to accommodate any fitness level and to adjust the exercise intensity during any segment of the workout.

Water also transfers exercise heat away from the body much more quickly than air at the same temperature. Pool temperatures between 80 and 84 degrees Fahrenheit (about 27 to 29 degrees Celsius) feel cool and refreshing, and you will find that you can tolerate longer workouts without feeling overheated. Longer workouts use more energy and provide greater overall fitness results.

Improving and Maintaining Fitness

If you were to perform an exercise in the water at the same speed as you can on land, you would find it nearly impossible to keep pace. This is because water has so much more resistance than air. Research has shown that water, if manipulated with purpose, is heavy enough to create an overload to improve heart health, build muscular endurance, and in some cases improve muscular strength. You can also improve flexibility in opposing muscle groups just by maintaining a functional range of motion throughout the workout. People who have worked out in the water, whether swimming or water fitness, report that they have improved their muscle tone, strengthened their core muscles, and improved their flexibility. Many people also report that they have lost weight and slimmed down. This too is supported by research. The energy expended in water workouts helps maintain body weight or improve body composition, especially when combined with healthy dietary adjustments.

Keeping Fun in Fitness

The consequences of a sedentary lifestyle are evidenced in the number of deaths attributed to cardiovascular diseases and the ever-increasing reports on the childhood obesity epidemic in the United States. To combat this, fitness activities should be encouraged and included in the lifestyles of young people. This is, at times, a difficult task because workouts can seem like punishment or drudgery. However, exercising in the water can be an exhilarating experience. Water that is clean, clear, and sparkling is enticing and refreshing. Add fun and games to the workout plan and your participants will be excited, laughing, pleasantly surprised, and willing to come back again. They will discover that they can do many things that they cannot do on land. They can do kickboxing or martial arts without falling. They can try jumps and bounding activities that would normally create too much impact for knees and ankles. They can also run around and play games that become more challenging in the water without the added risks of injury.

Water workouts have a social and emotional component as well. Water equalizes play because it is a foreign environment for everyone and almost all can participate in some fashion. It doesn't matter who is on which team because everyone has the same "disadvantage." Participation in interactive water games promotes self-esteem and provides opportunities to establish new friendships. Participants have the opportunity to forget the stresses of the day, play hard, and go home happy. And this is only the beginning.

Swimming: A Life Skill

Experiencing water and water games in a standing position where submersion is not required builds confidence and reduces fear. As participants experience and learn to trust buoyancy during games and activities, they will be more willing to float and paddle in the horizontal position. In fact, they will find swimming mechanics easier and faster when playing tag games and participating in relay events. These experiences make the next steps of learning to swim less threatening and much simpler.

Swimming is a life skill and a personal safety skill. It opens doors to dozens of new and different aquatic activities that can be enjoyed with family and friends while vacationing or just hanging out at the pool.

Swimming provides many of the same benefits as water fitness but is even gentler on the joints. As we age we often find it difficult to tolerate the stress of land-based exercise. Swimming is a wonderful alternative and can be enjoyed much later in life than many other sports. In addition, there are opportunities to compete in Masters meets (over age 19) and senior (over age 50) swimming events all over the world. Swimming in competition later in life provides a needed social outlet and helps improve the quality of life.

As you can see, there are many reasons to introduce water fitness and swimming skills into your program. What better way to combat the creeping obesity epidemic than to provide a fitness outlet that is easy on the joints, doesn't cause heat stress, and is fun and exhilarating! Most important, by incorporating fun in water fitness, you have the opportunity to encourage a fitness habit and to promote aquatic skills that will ultimately help people develop a valuable life skill. Go for it!

chapter 2

Activity Selection and Modifications

Selecting activities for your group begins with observing participants to see what abilities they have and how comfortable they feel in the water. The Fitness Activity Finder (pages vii to ix) provides a quick way to locate activities suitable for warm-up or cool-down, cardiorespiratory endurance training, and interval training. In this chapter we'll also briefly discuss how to modify activities for people with disabilities and how to use equipment to make workouts more fun and effective.

Although selecting fitness activities is the focus of this chapter, once participants master the basics they can easily make the transition from water exercise to swimming. The Swim Activity Finder on pages x to xi helps you easily locate appropriate swimming skills and games that work best for your group. (See chapter 6 for more information on selecting swim activities.)

Testing for Readiness

Everyone who can move independently around the pool in shallow water can participate in water workouts, water games that train (presented in chapter 5), and skills that prepare you to learn to swim (presented in chapter 6). Balance may be an issue for some, but coordination should not be a problem because the water slows movement and makes it easier to execute skills. The easiest way to determine what activities will work for your group is to test participants in the water on independent locomotor skills.

Have participants experiment in water no more than chest deep. Deeper water reduces traction and makes it more difficult to move across the playing area. In addition, participants will experience more buoyancy when the water is deeper, and this may make apprehensive participants fearful or uncomfortable.

Have participants warm up by traveling back and forth across the pool demonstrating the following independent locomotor skills, using the arms for balance.

- Walking
- Jogging
- Jumping off one foot
- Hopping (two feet)
- Skipping
- Leaping
- Stepping sideways

Notice how each participant performs the skill. Does anyone struggle with balance? Do some seem uncomfortable as the water approaches chest deep, or spread their arms out wide to maintain balance or keep their hands moving in an attempt to stay upright? These are all signs of apprehension. Try pairing these folks with a partner who has experience in the water, or allow them to stay near a wall during play.

Participants who are apprehensive should be taught how to get their feet back underneath them in the event that they fall off balance during a game or activity. This skill is called *recovery to a stand* and is described in detail in chapter 3 (page 27).

Using the Fitness Activity Finder

The fitness activity finder at the front of this book is organized so that you can quickly identify activities in chapters 4 and 5 that will help you reach your fitness goals. The types of activity in the finder include the following:

- **Arm works**—Activities that isolate the arm muscles for muscular endurance or, if equipment is used, for strength training. Arm works are combined with independent locomotion to create the aqua basic building blocks.
- **Aqua basics**—Combinations of independent locomotor skills and arm works that are the building blocks for a variety of workouts. Once participants are able to successfully perform these skills, these building blocks can be incorporated into game play.
- **Sport aqua**—Exercises that are commonly used to train for land-based activities such as tennis, volleyball, basketball, cheerleading, and kickboxing.
- **Partner stunts and skills**—Stunts and skills broaden the workout options. They are activities that pair individuals of like size, strength, and abilities to complete a task. They are described early in chapter 5 so that they can be used in variations of game play.
- **Relay games**—Variations of the shuttle relay format (described in chapter 5).
- **Tag games**—Variations of games in which a person or persons designated as "It" chase and contact or capture other participants, making their roles in the game change.
- **Individual events**—Activities that one person can do to enhance fitness. These are easily incorporated into a workout plan.
- **Team events**—Activities played by groups of individuals forming a team and having a competitive objective. These are often used as part of the interval training within the workout design because participants are willing to work harder to win the game.

The fitness focus column indicates which activities are appropriate for the fitness goals or particular section of any workout. For example, any warm-up and cool-down activities listed in this section will help prepare the participant for the harder work ahead (or cool down after doing that harder work). Many of the games can be modified slightly to transition from warm-up to cardiorespiratory endurance, and then to interval sets within the same game. Generally, the adaptation simply requires moving slowly at first, increasing speed to a "steady-state" mode for cardiorespiratory endurance, and then combining a high-intensity repeat with a recovery phase to create the interval sets.

Let's take a few moments to define the components that appear in the fitness focus:

- Warm-up and cool-down
- Cardiorespiratory endurance
- Interval training
- Muscular endurance

Warm-Up and Cool-Down

Warm-up and cool-down activities can take many forms. They are grouped together in this section because all that is necessary to change a warm-up activity to a cool-down activity is to reverse the progression. In other words, the warm-up slowly builds intensity for the first 5 to 10 minutes of the workout, whereas the cool-down slowly decreases the intensity for the last 5 to 10 minutes of the workout. With few exceptions, these same activities work equally well for both parts of the workout.

Warm-up activities are performed in slow motion, using active range of motion to stretch opposing muscle groups. Static stretching isn't necessary at this time because participants are not warm enough to keep from becoming chilly if they have to stand still. Warm-up activities are a great time to introduce participants to the new skill challenges that will be repeated later in the workout. It is an opportunity to get participants focused on posture and good body mechanics and to help them get comfortable with a skill element. Once they have warmed up with proper mechanics, they will be able to add speed and energy with limited risk of injury.

Cool-down periods simply reverse the process of the warm-up. This is the appropriate time to incorporate static stretching. However, if the water is cold, participants may be able to tolerate only short periods of stretching. For this reason, you may not be able to address flexibility as a component of your program under these conditions.

Cardiorespiratory Endurance

Cardiorespiratory endurance (referring to cardiorespiratory fitness) is the ability of the body to deliver oxygen to the working muscles and to effectively use that oxygen. We can improve the cardiorespiratory system with periods of aerobic exercise and aerobic intervals. To realize benefits to the cardiorespiratory system, exercise must be moderate to vigorous. The American College of Sports Medicine (ACSM) recommends a minimum of 20 minutes of aerobic activity, or two or more bouts of at least 10 minutes.

For best results, any aerobic exercise program should comply with the recommendations provided by ACSM and follow the FIT formula:

Frequency—How often? (3 to 5 times per week)

Intensity—How hard? (60 to 80 percent of heart rate reserve)

Time—How long per workout? (20 to 60 minutes)

The most important variable is the intensity of the workout. The intensity of the aerobic set is determined by calculating a percentage of the heart rate or by assessing your perception of how hard you are working (also referred to as *rating of perceived exertion,* or RPE). To figure a heart rate necessary for improvements in the cardiorespiratory system, use the heart rate reserve (HRR) formula shown in figure 2.1.

Figuring Target Heart Rate

Use this formula to figure target heart rate using the heart rate reserve method.

1. Subtract your age from 220.

   220 − age = ___ (A)

2. Determine your resting heart rate (RHR). Sit quietly for 10 minutes, then take a pulse count for 1 full minute. This is your resting heart rate (RHR).

   RHR = ___

3. Subtract your RHR from (A) in step 1.

   A − RHR = ___ (B)

4. Multiply (B) by 60% intensity (.60).

   B × .60 = ___ (C)

5. Add RHR from step 2 to (C) from step 4 to get the lower limit of the target heart rate zone.

   C + RHR = ___

6. Repeat steps 4 and 5 using 80% intensity (.80) to find the upper limit of the target heart rate zone.

Figure 2.1   Figure a target heart rate using the heart rate reserve method.

Have participants take a 6-second heart rate about every 10 minutes to determine whether they are working hard enough. Once they understand that the heart rate goes up when they work harder, teach them how to use an RPE scale. We recommend using a scale from 6 to 20. A rating of 6 means they are still sleeping, and 20 means they are being chased by a very hungry shark. You can use your creativity to give verbal cues for the other numbers, or use the RPE chart in figure 2.2 (see page 11). In general, on a scale from 6 to 20 you would want participants to be working at 13 to 15, or what would be considered "somewhat hard" to "hard."

The simplest way to work into the cardiorespiratory endurance set is to speed up the warm-up activities a little until the class begins to breathe a little harder. You can start with the aqua basics described in chapter 4 and then use your creativity, your coaching background, or your favorite physical activity to develop patterns or themes for continuing the workout. Sample patterns and workout designs appear at the end of chapters 4 and 5.

Interval Training

There's more than one way to improve the cardiorespiratory system. A very efficient way is to incorporate aerobic intervals into the workout. That is where the higher-intensity activities and the tag games and relay games fit in. They challenge the heart at a higher intensity, then include

Aqua Heart Rates

There is an ongoing controversy about the use of heart rates to monitor exercise intensity in the water. Because of the many factors that affect heart rate in the water, it is difficult to compare the existing research and come to a definite conclusion on whether to use heart rates. Though a complete review of research is beyond the scope of this book, we can offer a brief perspective of what current research implies.

For the most part, heart rates will decrease under the following conditions:

- In cooler water (82 degrees Fahrenheit or 27.8 degrees Celsius, or less; conflicting evidence in water greater than 83 degrees Fahrenheit or 28.3 degrees Celsius)
- As depth increases (heart rates are consistently lower in water from nipple deep to the neck)
- As exercise protocols call for maximum exertion (heart rates are consistently lower at maximum levels)
- With the participants' lack of skill or motivation to produce the necessary effort
- As the style of the workout includes more curved movements, bouncing, and reliance on buoyancy

In addition to these variables, no one has even looked at the effect of acclimation over time and its effect on heart rates in the water.

While most advise reducing target heart rates by 10 to 15 beats below the land-based heart rate reserve figures to accommodate these changes, a closer look reveals several flaws in that thinking. First, most of us will not exercise in water at a temperature below about 84 degrees Fahrenheit (about 29 degrees Celsius). In addition, this and most shallow-water programs recommend water depths from the navel to the nipple line. Finally, with so many different exercise protocols, skill levels, and motivational levels, one might underestimate a target zone and reduce cardiorespiratory results.

That said, we recommend that you not manipulate the land-based heart rate reserve method but rather use it in combination with a rating of perceived exertion for comparison in order not to underestimate the target zone and lose results.

For a complete review of related research and recommendations, see chapter 1 of *Aquatic Fitness, Everyone* (2005) by Terri Lees.

a resting period between games. Cardiorespiratory endurance and intervals are listed separately in the fitness focus column to distinguish a higher work effort.

A complete discussion of interval training is beyond the scope of this book, but basically exercise can be done in intervals to enhance both cardiorespiratory endurance and sprinting ability. The benefits of interval training are well documented. Interval training allows more work to be done in less time than continuous training.

For ease of discussion, let's define a few terms related to interval training:

- **Exercise interval**—Refers to the length (in seconds) of the work phase being performed during each repetition.
- **Interval set**—Refers to a group of repetitions.
- **Relief or recovery phase**— Refers to the length of time (in seconds) of the rest between repetitions or sets. Relief or recovery phases can be *active recovery* or *rest recovery*.
- **Active recovery phase**—During this phase, you continue to move gently, walking, slowly jogging, or performing other basic exercises between the repetitions and between the sets. This is appropriate for the recovery interval during cardiorespiratory endurance interval training. The length in seconds of the active recovery should be no longer than one-quarter to one-third the length in seconds of the work or exercise interval.
- **Rest recovery phase**—Refers to inactive resting; in other words, you relax and float instead of moving. This type of recovery phase is most appropriate for sprint-type anaerobic training. The length of the rest recovery phase is determined by the intensity of the work phase. In general, the greater the intensity of the sprint work, the

6	No exertion at all
7	
	Extremely light
8	
9	Very light
10	
11	Light
12	
13	Somewhat hard
14	
15	Hard (heavy)
16	
17	Very hard
18	
19	Extremely hard
20	Maximal exertion

Figure 2.2 Use the Borg Scale in combination with a target heart rate to monitor your intensity.

Reprinted, by permission, from G. Borg, 1998, *Borg's perceived exertion and pain scales* (Champaign, IL: Human Kinetics), 47.

© Gunnar Borg, 1970, 1985, 1994, 1998

longer the rest recovery. At a minimum, the rest recovery in seconds should equal the duration of the work in seconds. At higher intensities, rest recovery can and should be as much as four times the work interval.

- **Repetition or cycle**—Refers to the completion of a predetermined amount of work (for the purpose of this discussion given in seconds or minutes) and includes both the exercise or work phase and the relief or recovery phase.
- **Series**—Refers to a group of sets, including the recovery phase.

Interval sets established for cardiorespiratory endurance will have a duration of at least 3 minutes of exercise followed by active recovery. To design your interval sets, you will have to determine the following:

1. Goal of the interval set or series (cardiorespiratory endurance or sprint training)
2. Length of the exercise interval (work phase)
3. Length of the relief phase and the type of relief (active or rest)
4. Type of active recovery, if applicable (for example, jog between repetitions, easy jumping jacks between sets)
5. Number of sets
6. Length and type of relief phase needed to do multiple sets (a series)
7. Type of relief between sets

Consider the following example, assuming an adequate warm-up:

Goal: Cardiorespiratory endurance

Exercise interval: 45 seconds (working somewhat hard to hard)

Relief phase: 15 seconds (one-third of the exercise interval)

Type of relief: Active recovery (jogging between repetitions)

Repetition: 1 minute

Number of repetitions: 10 (for this example, 5 repetitions for each leg using side kicks)

Length of the set: 10 minutes

In this example participants kick for 45 seconds, jog easily for 15 seconds, then repeat the kick, alternating right and left legs with each repetition. Ten minutes of the same activity continuously would be too stressful, but because of the active recovery participants can sustain the repeated activity. However, instead of doing a series of sets, you should probably select exercise combinations that allow total rest of the muscles used in kicking. For example, you might follow this set with a punching set lasting 3 to 5 minutes.

The fun begins when you start using tag games and relays to establish the repetitions within each interval set. Consider the following example, again assuming that you have provided an adequate warm-up:

Goal 1: Cardiorespiratory endurance

Exercise interval: 1 minute (working somewhat hard)

Relief phase: 15 seconds

Type of relief: Active recovery (skipping rope between sets)

Repetition: 1 minute, 15 seconds

Number of repetitions: 5 (alternating games for the duration of the exercise and then skipping back to the starting point)

Length of set: 6 minutes, 15 seconds

Goal 2: Sprint training

Exercise interval: 15 to 30 seconds (depending on the size of the playing area; working hard to very hard)

Relief phase: 45 to 90 seconds (for example, during a relay race everyone waits for a turn)

Type of relief: Rest recovery (float or rest on back)

Repetition: Approximately 1 to 2 minutes per participant

Number of repetitions: 3 to 5

Length of set: 3 to 10 minutes

Many tag games are perfect for high-energy cardiorespiratory endurance interval training. Be sure that everyone keeps moving to keep the intensity up during the work phase. For example, for goal 1, combine repetitions of Fusion Tag with Follow the Leader. For goal 2, use combinations of relay races to allow for more rest.

If you want to work on sport conditioning that involves high-intensity, longer-rest repeats, you can increase the intensity and shorten the length of the work phase to between 10 and 90 seconds and lengthen the rest recovery phase so that you can do the repeats at a similar intensity each time. For example, have participants perform a high-intensity game or activity for the work phase, then rest, relax, and float during the recovery phase.

Muscular Endurance

An added benefit of cardiorespiratory endurance and interval sets is the overall improvement in muscular endurance. Muscular endurance is the ability to repeat a movement, skill, or activity over and over again with little or no fatigue, such as lifting boxes onto a truck all day or carrying groceries to cars for hours at a time. These activities and many other daily living skills require muscular endurance. Because water is so heavy, movements in the cardiorespiratory endurance set have the potential to overload the muscles and improve muscular endurance. Developing muscular endurance, then, is simply a matter of working the water with purpose during the cardiorespiratory endurance set or when isolating specific muscle groups. Improvements are possible because all that is required is low resistance (water weight) and multiple repetitions over time. You will find that most of the activity objectives include muscular endurance for specific muscle groups.

In addition to muscular endurance, there is a potential to improve strength in certain muscle groups during the cardiorespiratory endurance and interval portions of the workout. However, because strength improvements are possible only with heavy loads (minimum of 60 percent of a one-repetition max), a relatively fit population may need additional equipment to create an effective workload. Because of budget constraints in many school and recreational programs, we have chosen not to discuss the development of muscular strength at this time but will include more information at the end of the chapter (see "Using Equipment to Enhance Play," page 15).

Adapting Games and Stunts for Individual Needs

The Americans with Disabilities Act and similar legislation encourage the inclusion of individuals with disabilities into regular classes. It is likely that you will have people with special needs in your class, group, or program. Do not assume that all such individuals need special adaptations, especially in the aquatic setting. The buoyancy of the water supports movement and gives many people with noticeable disabilities the freedom to move independently. Before providing adaptations for your participants with disabilities, give them the opportunity to try the skills involved in the activity. If they are unsuccessful, you will have some idea of their personal abilities and can adjust the game or stunt accordingly. The following information provides you with some options for adapting games to fit your participants.

- *Change or simplify the rules.* Younger participants need less complex rules to understand and enjoy the games. Make the game simple or change a rule that would make it difficult for someone with a disability to participate. When doing fitness games that require vertical posture, allow individuals with disabilities to use a horizontal posture more like swimming to reduce resistance and give them a slight advantage.

- *Change the size of the area.* Make the play area smaller for less advanced participants. Use the whole pool for more advanced groups.

- *Use a different depth of water or various depths.* Set up the game so that individuals with disabilities can be in shallower water to improve traction. Move a deep-water game to chest-deep water and do not allow swimmers to swim. Challenge participants who can swim by requiring that they play in deep water only. Use all areas of the pool.

- *Have all participants wear a life jacket or participate with a pool noodle or other buoyant device.* Be sure that everyone is comfortable with a life jacket on and can perform a simple swimming stroke well enough to return to the side of the pool independently in both shallow and deep water. If using noodles, do not allow nonswimmers into deep water using only a noodle for support. You can use the whole pool area and make the game fun for nonswimmers, yet challenging for better swimmers. Individuals with disabilities can use the life jacket or another buoyancy device to assist standing posture in shallow water. A noodle is perfect for assisting walking balance.

- *Provide a handicap for participants without disabilities.* Make them hold on to a piece of equipment like a noodle or a kickboard to slow them down during a fast-paced game. Or instruct them to keep their hands on their hips so that they cannot use their arms to help them travel. You might have stronger, more experienced participants wear sweatshirts or tie one arm to their side to slow them down, or let them swim or travel using only one arm. In games that require hitting, throwing, or catching a ball, you could strap oven mitts on more experienced ball handlers. You can also challenge them by allowing them to propel themselves only by kicking or jogging without their arms assisting while letting others swim. Jogging or kicking is much less efficient than swimming strokes.

- *Pair individuals with disabilities with participants without disabilities.* In many of the buddy stunts, individuals with a disability or nonswimmers can be paired successfully with an individual who swims well or has no disability. When using any of these suggestions, be sure to change partners frequently, either during a break in the game or between games, to improve tolerance and social interaction among the students.

Using Equipment to Enhance Play

Equipment can add a new dimension to a water activity class. Most pools have certain equipment such as kickboards and noodles that are readily available to all users. Other facilities may have fins, hand paddles, and other training equipment available as well. If your budget does not allow you to purchase pool play equipment, look in your fitness class supplies and see what equipment you can adapt for the pool. Many balls, including golf balls and rubber sport balls, can increase poolside enjoyment. Wiffle ball equipment can also be used successfully in the pool area.

There are a number of different reasons to add equipment to the workout. Most equipment increases the challenge to balance, stability, and muscle strength and endurance. Equipment can be used with intervals, relays, and team games to enhance play or to equalize individual or team efforts in an effort to keep the game fair.

Another important reason to add equipment is for the joy of playing and exploring new alternatives to basic skills. You will find kickboard stunts and noodle activities that are challenging to individuals and at times require partners to figure out the best and fastest way to manipulate the equipment to improve play. Sometimes the attempts at stunts with equipment are hysterically funny, and you find your participants laughing with each other because they all look goofy. Some of the activities in each area are probably more fun than they are functional, but we hope that you understand the importance of incorporating fun into fitness.

If you want more information about equipment and equipment safety, refer to appendix A. Appendix B provides a resource list for pool and play equipment. If equipment is an option to add to a game or activity, it will be indicated on the Fitness Activity Finder. However, you will need to consult the specific game to determine what equipment is necessary and whether you have enough equipment for a variation of the game or activity.

You should now have a good idea of how to select activities for the participants in your class. Assess the abilities and needs of your participants, and then find appropriate activities in the Fitness Activity Finder. When necessary, adapt those activities for individuals. Also use equipment to make your workouts more effective, as well as to add variety and fun to your classes.

chapter 3

Aquatic Program Safety

Safety is a major concern in an aquatic program. Safe water activities require good organization and risk management planning. Risk management is a process of identifying and managing the risks of an activity with the intent of reducing the incidence of injury to the participants. It is a responsibility shared by facility operators, program supervisors, and instructors alike. Facility operators are responsible for facility safety and, in most cases, for the supervision of the patrons. Program supervisors and instructors must plan for safety during the activities and programs they conduct. Although the aquatic environment by its nature will always hold an element of risk, a comprehensive risk management plan can reduce the injury potential of aquatic activities. It's also vital to teach participants basic skills that will keep them safe as they use the pool. Finally, you, as the instructor, must also make sure that your duties don't unnecessarily expose you to health and safety risks.

IMPORTANT! Please note that although some rescue skills are described in this text, this information does not accredit anyone to do lifesaving or lifeguarding. The primary purpose of this text is to provide safe water exercises and lead-up activities for learning to swim.

Facility Safety

In most cases, the instructor or supervisor of a program does not have direct responsibility for the operation of the facility in which the program operates, but a safe program begins with a safe facility. Before the program begins, tour the facility you intend to use. Make certain that lifeguard supervision will be provided for your program. Check the facility for safety hazards. Look for clear, sparkling water; murky water can reduce visibility and hamper supervision.

The deck, locker room, and shower areas should have slip-resistant surfaces. There should be no areas where standing water can cause slips and falls. The deck and pool should also be free of obstructions. A safety line should divide the shallow area from the deep, and water depths should be clearly marked on the deck and vertical wall of the pool at different areas around the pool.

The facility safety checklist in table 3.1 provides additional information on the pool safety check. If you find areas of concern, bring them to the attention of the pool operator immediately. You will have to decide if the risks you have identified can be managed with good program and activity safety. If not, you may need to reconsider using the facility.

Program Safety

As you plan your program, be aware of aquatic activities that increase the chance of personal injury. Plan your program to eliminate or control these activities. The most dangerous activities and situations in a pool area are

- swimming underwater after hyperventilating;
- diving into shallow water;
- horseplay, especially dunking;
- unsupervised use of scuba equipment;
- overcrowding of the pool;
- tag games, especially if participants chase each other on the deck;
- playing Follow the Leader off the springboard; and
- unsupervised use of flotation devices.

Table 3.1   Facility Safety Checklist

	Yes	No
Pool deck		
Clean		
Slip-resistant surface		
Free of obstruction		
Comfortable temperature (air temperature should be about 2 to 3 degrees Fahrenheit, or about 1.5 degrees Celsius, above pool temperature)		
Depth markings		
Adequate lighting		
Electrical safety (outlets at least 10 feet from pool edge)		
Clear, visible signage		
Disability access		
Pool bottom		
Smooth surface		
Marked for depth perception		
Gentle slope toward the deep water		
Ladders		
Nonslip steps		
Securely attached to the deck		
Steps		
Handrails securely attached		
Nonslip steps		
Contrasting color to mark the edge of the step		
Locker rooms and showers		
Clean		
Slip-resistant floor		
Benches and lockers in good repair		
Good lighting		
Good drainage		

(continued)

Table 3.1   (continued)

	Yes	No
Pool water		
Clear, sparkling water		
Comfortable temperature		
No strong odor of chlorine		
Safety equipment (accessible and in good repair)		
Long reaching pole		
Ring buoy		
Backboard (including a head immobilizer)		
Line separating shallow from deep water		
First aid station		
Rules posted		
Telephone or other communication system		
Supervision		
Guard chairs (at least 5 feet, or 1.5 meters, high)		
Guards attentive, on duty		
Instructor supervision		
Appropriate class size		

Reprinted, by permission, from T. Lees, 2005, *Aquatic fitness everyone* (Winston-Salem, NC: Hunter Textbooks, Inc.), 310.

You can minimize the risks by providing good supervision, establishing and enforcing rules, and planning for possible emergencies.

Supervision

Your ability to adequately supervise an aquatic program depends a great deal on your professional training and that of other staff, as well as the instructor-to-student ratio. Ideally, a lifeguard should be supervising the activity. It is not enough for you to play both roles. The accepted standard of care for aquatic programs is that a certified lifeguard, with no other duties than to supervise patrons, should be on duty at all times during the activities. As you review the activities in this book, it will become obvious that more often than not, you will conduct the activity to keep the workout and game play going. This will not allow you to provide uninterrupted supervision of the participants.

All instructors should have credentials that indicate that they can teach in the aquatic area. (Associations that offer this training are listed in appendix C.) Lifeguards should be trained by a recognized agency, have good skills, and maintain current certificates in first aid, CPR, and the use of an AED and supplemental oxygen. Safety and rescue equipment should be available to the guards, who may need to respond to an incident or accident in the pool. Equipment available at the pool should include a rescue tube, a fanny pack with pocket mask and gloves, a backboard with straps, cervical collars and a head immobilizer, and access to an AED and supplemental oxygen. However, as equipment, rules, and regulations differ from state to state, you need to review your applicable codes to be certain that you are in compliance.

Even if your facility seems reasonably safe, you should still develop a regular pattern of inspection. Check the facility and equipment daily. Make sure that safety equipment and equipment for class activities is available and in good condition. Do not use faulty equipment. Report any hazards to management immediately, and if these hazards mean that you cannot conduct your program safely, cancel the class.

The facility size, the area of shallow water available, and the skill level of the group will affect how many students you can safely teach and supervise. Participants should have a personal workout space of at least 15 square feet (4.5 square meters) of surface area to accommodate active water fun and fitness games. Swimming activities require even more room. A position statement written for the Council for Aquatic Professionals of the American Alliance for Health, Physical Education, Recreation and Dance (AAHPERD) recommends that the instructor-to-student ratio not exceed 1 teacher for each 20 to 25 students. You may need to work creatively to keep larger groups rotating into and out of the activity areas.

You can improve your chances of maintaining a safe program if you involve the class or group in the safety of the program. First, establish a communication system. For example, one short whistle means everyone must freeze. Two short whistles means it's time for a buddy check. One long whistle means everyone must clear the pool. Three short whistles means participants should resume play.

Second, teach the participants the *buddy system*. Each person is assigned or may choose a buddy to keep track of during the activity. Each buddy pair has a number. On the signal (two short whistles) buddies clasp hands and hold them above their heads. As soon as the group is quiet, the buddy pairs count off, beginning with number one and continuing until all pairs have been counted. Any person who cannot locate his or her buddy during the class activity or for buddy check should report this to the lifeguard or instructor immediately. At this point you should clear the pool and begin a search.

Practicing buddy checks periodically throughout the program will increase your chances of successfully managing an emergency. One option is to have buddy pairs move immediately to the nearest wall and hop out before the count begins. This is also a great way to practice for a quick evacuation.

In addition to these safety measures, teach participants how to perform a basic water rescue to assist a buddy in case of an emergency. The simplest and safest forms of rescue are ones that do not put the rescuer in jeopardy. Participants can be taught to reach from the deck, to extend an arm or leg from in the water while holding on to the side, to wade with a noodle, and to assist another swimmer by helping the swimmer walk toward the exit in standing-depth water.

Call for Lifeguards First

Although you may choose to teach rescue skills to participants, please be sure to make it clear to them that if they see someone in the pool in trouble, they should alert the lifeguard on duty immediately. Even if participants know how to perform rescue skills, it's safer, especially for children, to have the trained lifeguard do the rescue. A panicked swimmer can be dangerous, particularly when the rescuer is also in the water.

- *Reach:* Lie down on the deck and spread the legs out to provide a wider base of support. Hold the deck securely with one hand and reach your other hand out to grasp the victim. Pull him slowly to the side of the pool.

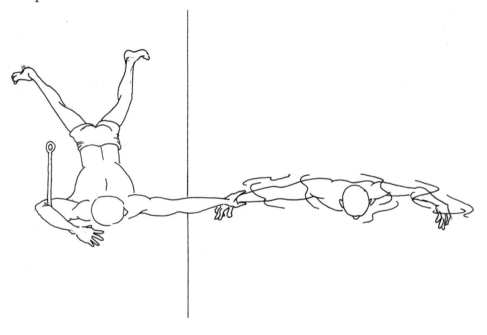

- *Extend:* If you cannot reach the victim from the deck, you may either extend a piece of equipment from the position just described or slide carefully into the pool and maintain a firm grasp on the side of the pool. Extend an arm or leg toward the victim. Slowly draw the victim toward you and the side of the pool.

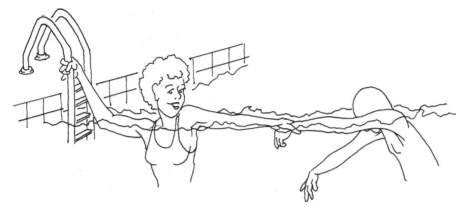

- *Wade with a noodle:* Never attempt a wading assist in water more than chest deep or in moving water. Keep a noodle extended in front of you and wade out until the victim can grab it. Slowly walk backward toward shallower water and bring the victim to the side.

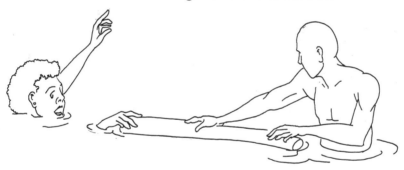

- *Walking assist:* If a person is not able to get back to his feet in standing-depth water, come to the side of the victim and grasp the closest arm, wrapping it around your neck for support. Reach your arm around the person's waist and help him get to his feet.

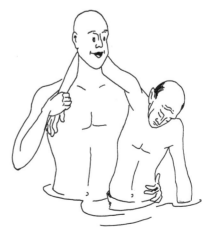

Rules and Policies

Establish and consistently enforce rules of the pool and any policies designed to support safety in programming. Your facility may have additional rules that are specific to the design of the pool. Provide a copy of the rules for each participant and take time in the first meeting to discuss the rules and reasons for each rule before entering the water. The following rules are considered standard precautions for aquatic safety:

- No running on the deck.
- No spitting or spouting in the pool.
- No horseplay on the deck.
- No pushing or shoving other swimmers into the pool.
- No diving into shallow water.

Some facilities have specific rules for the safe use or nonuse of flotation devices. A flotation device can be free floating, such as a noodle or a kickboard, or it can be an attached device, such as a buoyant belt or a Coast Guard–approved life jacket. Nonswimmers must never be allowed to venture into deep water using a free-floating device. If they lose their grip, it could lead to drowning. Nonswimmers should always wear a Coast Guard–approved life jacket in deep water. It is certainly appropriate, however, for good swimmers to use kickboards or noodles in the deep water to support play activities as long as they are adequately supervised.

You may also need to establish rules that govern safe play during the fitness games and activities, such as what is considered appropriate touching during a tag game, a no-dunking rule, and rules that limit use of the deck as a play area. In addition, never allow participants to chew gum during the class. Gum is easily inhaled in the excitement of the game and can obstruct the airway.

As a general rule, you should be aware of the health status of those participating in your classes. Your facility should ask participants to complete health screening forms before they can participate. You should also have a policy that requires participants to inform you of any change in health status, and you should be ready to enforce a no-swim policy for any of the following contraindications:

- Open wounds
- Infectious diseases
- Unstable blood pressure
- Bladder or bowel incontinence
- Fever over 100 degrees Fahrenheit (38 degrees Celsius)

Emergency Plans

Your facility should have emergency action plans (EAPs) to handle a variety of emergencies. However, you also should prepare your class for emergency situations. Be certain that your participants understand their role in emergency procedures. Discuss the emergency signal with the class (one long whistle means everyone must clear the pool). Practice evacuating the pool (much like a fire drill) so that everyone knows where to seek safety. Evacuation of the pool must be organized to avoid complicating rescue efforts. Discuss locker room behavior if the class must evacuate to the locker room while you manage the emergency. If your program involves young children, you will need to plan for adult supervision in the locker room because you will likely have to handle the emergency in the pool area.

In addition, be sure the facility has an established plan for evacuation during an electrical storm and a protocol for dealing with vomit, solid stool, or a loose fecal accident in the pool. Check also to see if the facility has plans for managing medical or catastrophic emergencies and determine what role you should play, if any.

Table 3.2 is a checklist for program safety. Use it to ensure you have taken all the appropriate precautions to make your program safe for participants.

Participant Personal Safety

Learning personal safety skills as part of a water activities class will help increase participants' independence in the water. Personal safety skills also provide a necessary basis for stroke and stunt learning. Students who master the skills of entry and exit, recovery to a stand, and wearing a life jacket will be more relaxed in the water and will enjoy a variety of games and stunts.

Independent Entry and Exit

Participants should learn how to enter and exit the water independently and safely. Depending on your facility, this may mean walking down a ramp or sitting on the poolside and sliding into the water. Ladders should be used for exit only, as descending a ladder into the pool is not the safest approach.

Teach participants to use a jump entry into chest-deep water and to regain a balanced position. The feetfirst jump entry is recommended for entry into both shallow and deep water. The entry is much like the "compact jump" taught in lifeguarding. Have participants cross their arms over the chest and enter with the feet flat.

Table 3.2   Program Safety Checklist

Component	Considerations
Supervision	____ Instructor has training in basic water rescue. ____ Lifeguards are trained and certified by a nationally recognized agency. ____ Lifeguards are equipped with safety and rescue equipment. ____ Other rescue equipment is on deck or readily available. ____ Lifeguard supervision is available at all times. ____ An appropriate instructor–participant ratio (not to exceed 1 per 25 participants) is maintained. ____ Additional lifeguard supervision is provided if the size of the group exceeds the recommended ratio. ____ Participants are trained using a buddy system or equivalent process.
Policies and rules for participation	____ Safety rules are posted in the locker rooms before participants enter the pool area. ____ Rules are posted in the pool area. ____ Rules have been discussed with participants. ____ Instructor documents safety procedures for workouts and game play in the lesson plan. ____ A no-swim policy has been established for certain health conditions. ____ A return-to-activity policy has been established to state when participants who weren't permitted in class because of health conditions can return. ____ Rules are consistently enforced by the lifeguards and instructors. ____ Consequences for breaking the rules or for unsafe participation exist and are implemented.
Planning for emergencies	____ The facility has an emergency communication system. ____ Phone numbers for emergency assistance are prominently displayed near the phone. ____ An emergency script that lists the name and the address of the facility is posted near the phone. ____ The instructor has been educated about the emergency action plan. ____ There is a designated entrance for emergency personnel. ____ Participants have been educated about their personal behavior in the event of an emergency. ____ Lifeguards and other key support personnel have been thoroughly trained on managing an emergency.

From T. Lees, 2007, *Water fun* (Champaign, IL: Human Kinetics).

Jumping into deep water requires more advanced swimming skills. Lead-up skills are listed in chapter 6; consult them when your participants decide they are ready for this challenge.

Note that better swimmers enjoy using a headfirst or diving entry. However, diving into shallow water is a leading cause of spinal injury (in particular, broken necks). Do not allow students to dive into water shallower than 9 feet (about 3 meters). Do not teach diving if you have not received proper training in teaching diving progressions, and if there is a 1 meter board in the facility, do not allow diving from it unless the water under the board is a minimum of 11.5 feet (3.5 meters) deep.

Recovery to a Stand

This is a skill that participants who can swim do naturally. However, apprehensive participants may be caught off guard and may not be able to get their feet back under them when buoyancy takes over. Have participants practice a lead-up skill and then try the skill with the assistance of a partner. A noodle works well for the prone (front) position but not for the supine (back) position.

• *Lead-up (prone position):* Stand facing the wall and place both hands on the deck edge (coping) of the pool. Extend the legs behind so that you are in a diagonal position with the feet still on the bottom. Pull down on the wall and, at the same time, draw the knees up to the chest. Once the knees are beneath your shoulders, simply stand up.

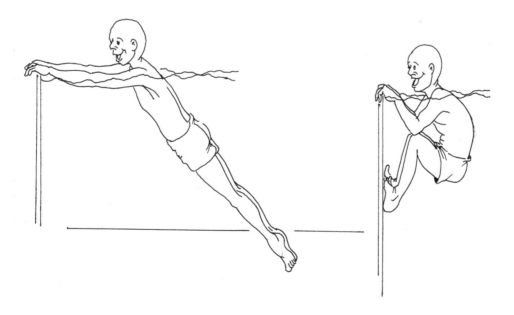

- *Lead-up with the noodle:* Grab the noodle and extend your arms in front of you as you glide slightly forward. Pull down on the noodle and, at the same time, pull the knees up toward the chin and continue as described previously.

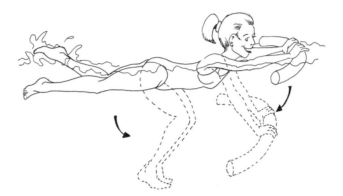

- *Assist to a stand (prone) with a partner assist:* Face your partner and, without submerging your head, reach your arms forward and glide slightly. As soon as your feet leave the bottom of the pool, pull down on the water and simultaneously pull the knees toward the chin. If you have difficulty, your partner is in position to grab your hands and assist you to a stand.

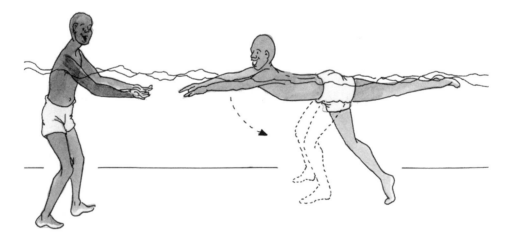

- *Assist to a stand (supine) with a partner assist:* Facing the wall, grab the wall with both hands and bend the knees to place the feet on the wall about hip high. Your partner stands behind you for support. Gently release the wall and push to a reclining position. As you feel your feet leave the wall, reach your arms behind you under the water and pull the water forward as you would if you were trying to pull a chair up to sit down. At the same time, curl the knees toward the chest and stick your

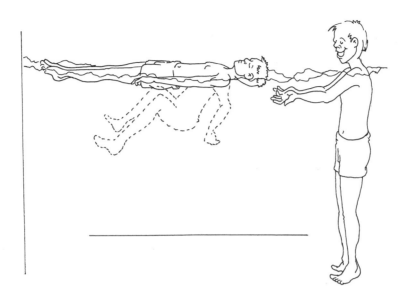

chin forward. The pull of your arms will allow you to quickly rotate into a vertical position, and then you stand up. Your partner can press against your back to help you recover if necessary.

Life Jacket Use

If life jackets are available, participants should know how to use them properly. Life jackets provide support for swimmers and nonswimmers alike. Life jackets should be U.S. Coast Guard approved and in good condition. Participants should be capable of donning a life jacket on deck and in shallow water. They should be able to perform a few swimming strokes on their front or back in order to be comfortable and independent. When entering the water using a life jacket, cross the arms over the chest and hold the life jacket down. Enter with the feet first and with the knees bent and the feet flat.

When teaching use of a life jacket, have participants practice in shallow water. If they cannot manage their body position or swim safely to the side in shallow water, they will not be able to experiment in deep water. Continued practice will be beneficial.

In addition to using life jackets, there are some other personal safety tips that should be taken into consideration:

- Maintain good hydration. Drink water before, during, and after exercise.
- If the program is conducted outdoors, wear sun protection such as sunscreen, sunglasses, or a broad-brimmed hat.
- For foot protection and slip resistance, purchase comfortable aqua shoes.

Instructor Safety

Teaching in an aquatic environment is truly a challenge, even for instructors who are in top shape. Instructors must spend time on a concrete or tile deck demonstrating and explaining movement. Neither surface provides for the kind of shock absorption needed to reduce impact stress on the joints. You must also deal with an environment that is much warmer than a gym or cooler outdoors during the spring and fall, and you will struggle to be heard if the facility has bad acoustics. Not paying attention to these issues may lead to serious injury and limit your ability to teach or participate in class activities. The suggestions in table 3.3 are offered to assist you with your personal health in an aquatic area.

Safety is an ever-present concern in the aquatic environment. Even the most prudent instructor can run into problems that just cannot be resolved. There are several ways to protect yourself from the consequences of incidents and accidents that may happen in the aquatic area. These include purchasing professional liability insurance; maintaining copies of lesson plans, rules, and reports from your program; and following the advice given in this chapter. You might also want to check with the legal department in your organization and ask about the use of participant waivers. With the help of the facility manager and the participants in your program, you can reduce the chances of accidents and injuries in your program. As you continue reading the rest of this book, review the strategies in this chapter frequently to ensure that you remain vigilant. This will keep the fun happening and the injuries to a minimum.

Table 3.3 Personal Safety Considerations

For your safety	Considerations
Reduce joint stress	Teach in the water when possible. Wear supportive shoes. Exercise on a mat. Sit in a chair and demonstrate when possible. Limit high-intensity aerobic-style presentations of games or skills.
Reduce heat stress	Drink fluids before, during, and after class. Dress comfortably. Teach while in the water when appropriate.
Reduce vocal stress	Drink fluid before, during, and after class. Limit the use of caffeine and decongestants that can dry the throat. Invest in a sound system. When using music, put it to the side instead of directly behind you. Record your vocal cues on a tape in advance. Use hand signals and whistle signals creatively to limit speaking.

chapter 4

Water Fitness Activities and Workouts

The activities in this chapter are the building blocks for water fun and fitness workouts and are appropriate for all parts of the workout as long as the intensity is adjusted to match your fitness goals. Begin all workouts with a slow warm-up of 5 to 10 minutes, and include range-of-motion activities to prepare the joints for the work ahead. Work into a cardiorespiratory endurance set with more intense "basics," then follow with games that train to create interval sets. Finish with a cool-down and a period of stretching.

We start by looking at the various ways you can use the water to increase resistance and create a more challenging workout. Then we review basic arm movements that can be combined with leg movements to create aqua basic activities. We present some specific activities appropriate for athletes in the sport aqua section, then finish the chapter with sample workout designs you can use with your program participants.

Effective Water Use

In order to make a safe transition from the warm-up to the intervals, you need to know how to work the water. The underlying principles of aquatic exercise are beyond the scope of this book, but a brief overview will help you understand how to manipulate the water and progressively increase the difficulty of the work and set the stage for interval games. Let's look at

- depth of water,
- body position,
- speed,
- range of motion,
- surface area or leverage,
- type of movement,
- effort, and
- progression.

- *Depth of water.* The activities in the basic workout and many of the games are more effective when performed in water that is approximately chest deep. Deeper water makes it more difficult to travel and allows participants to float more than they work. Position participants in chest-deep water for the best experience. When standing erect, they should have the water at the lower part of the sternum. For games, you are at the mercy of the pool design. Your play area may slope toward deeper water, and participants will need to move from shallow to deeper water in order to play.

Chest-deep water is best for executing arm works as well. Have participants bend their knees to submerge the arms a little deeper and take advantage of leverage. If you add buoyant equipment, like a kickboard or noodle, participants will need to be in water a little shallower (between the chest and the navel) to keep from floating off the bottom during the arm works.

- *Body position.* Working in a vertical position, especially traveling around the play area, is the best way to increase the drag, or resistance, during the workout. Ask participants to stand up straight and keep the shoulders over the hips. Leaning forward can cause them to float through the workout, especially when they bounce on their toes as in land-based activities. Bouncing and bounding from step to step are acceptable and fun, but they include a float phase that reduces intensity.

- *Speed.* Speed is probably the easiest way to increase the intensity of the cardiorespiratory endurance and interval sets. Moving faster increases the resistance exponentially. More resistance means that the muscles must work harder to complete the movement. It is fun to put the basics to music in order to maintain speed, especially if you have a theme to work with. If you use music, be sure to try the exercises in the water before presenting them to the class. Music between 100 and 125 beats per minute works well if you want to stay on beat. However, be careful not to reduce the range of motion too much to stay with the music, or participants will not be able to maintain intensity and use the muscles throughout their functional range of motion. Read on to see why.

- *Range of motion.* The bigger the move—for example, kicking hip high as opposed to kicking just off the floor—the more resistance you feel. The end of the limb (hand or foot) actually travels a farther distance in the same amount of time than the part of the limb nearest the joint. As a consequence, the hand or foot accelerates through the move. Remember that speed increases the resistance exponentially, so range of motion has a significant impact on the intensity and resistance.

- *Surface area or leverage.* Larger surface areas (or longer levers) increase resistance to movement. The difference in effort required to perform arm works with your hand open instead of a fist is incredible. The same happens when you lift your leg to kick as opposed to lifting your leg with your knee bent as when jogging (when speed and range of motion are held constant).

- *Type of movement.* Angles (movements in a straight line, back and forth) require more effort than curves (circular movements of the limbs). This is a fact swimmers have always known. They use curved movement patterns to increase force and reduce effort. So if you want to work harder, keep the arms and legs moving back and forth in a straight line.

- *Effort.* On land, each exercise that you perform has a power phase and a recovery phase. In the power phase you exert an effort to shorten the muscles and create the first part of the movement. In the recovery phase you simply return to the starting position. Water provides multi-dimensional resistance. You can emphasize power in one direction at a time and allow your body to relax as it returns (recovers to the starting position), or you can emphasize power in both directions. For example, you can work the biceps muscle by doing elbow flexion, palm open, and pulling the water toward the surface (power up). You work the triceps by pulling the arm back to the starting position (power down; see figure 4.1 on page 36). While it is true that you should isolate a muscle group for strength training, during the cardiorespiratory endurance set you will get better results when you work hard in both directions, creating two power phases back to back. This can also save time over traditional

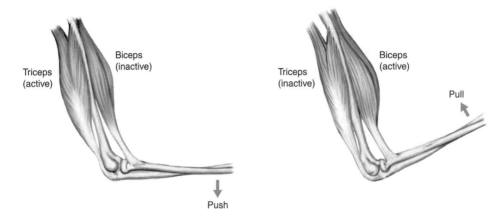

Figure 4.1   "Power down" for triceps and "power up" for biceps.

endurance workouts because you can improve muscular endurance in opposing muscle groups with the same exercise.

• *Progression.* Use an add-on approach with the other variables that affect intensity. Add speed, then range of motion, then longer levers, then straight-line movement, and then perform your power phases in both directions and watch how the work becomes harder. Once you have experienced these options, try traveling. Move forward, backward, to the side, or in a circle and experiment with the power of moving water when you stop, start, speed up, slow down, or change directions. The moving water behind you creates additional resistance that you can manipulate as you work arms and legs to isolate specific muscle groups.

Arm Works

The arm motions are described first in this chapter for several reasons. First, they will be paired with the legs in the next section to create the aqua basics building blocks for workout design. Second, the resistance of the water during movements leads to local muscular fatigue. As you begin to tire out, you will be forced to reduce the intensity in some way or stop altogether to rest. One way to extend the duration of the cardiorespiratory endurance set is to change the muscles you are working. For example, when the legs get tired and heavy, stop in place and do repeats of the arm works. This keeps the core muscles (specifically, abdominal and lower-back muscles) engaged and helps overload for specific upper-body muscular endurance.

When you isolate the arms, always assume a proper lifting stance. The back should be straight, with shoulders in line over the hips. Feet should be shoulder-width apart and knees bent to submerge to the depth of about the armpits. Keep the core area (abdomen and lower back muscles) tight as you lift. Establish a regular pattern of breathing, exhaling on the power phase and inhaling on the recovery phase or return to the starting position. Do not hold your breath.

SWIM STROKES

Objectives Stroking; muscular endurance in the upper back (trapezius), back upper arm (triceps), and midback (latissimus dorsi)

Description Stand in a stride or straddle position.

Breaststroke: Begin with arms extended in front of the body (shoulder flexion) on the surface of the water. Pull arms back simultaneously, bending the elbows to point the palms back. Recover the arms close to the body and return to the starting position.

Front crawl: Use an arm-over-arm stroke to reach forward and down into the water and pull back to a position behind the body (pretend to pass one handful of water at a time to someone behind you). Arms may recover over or under the water.

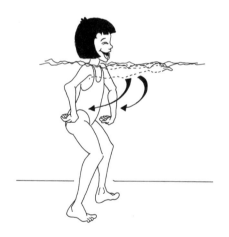 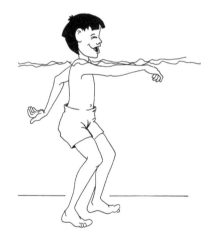

Variation

Pass the Splash: Form a circle with participants turned to the side so that they have the right or left shoulder to the center of the circle (all are facing the same direction and facing someone's back). All practice the swimming strokes by "passing the splash" to the person behind them. This encourages finishing the pull and will be valuable as participants learn to swim.

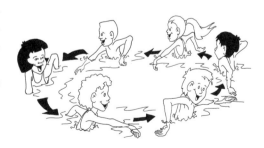

BUTTERFLY

Objectives
Stretching; muscular endurance in the upper chest (pectoralis, power phase forward) and upper back (trapezius, power phase backward)

Description
Extend arms out to the side (shoulder abduction). Bend elbows slightly and point them to the bottom of the pool. Face palms in, thumbs up. Pull the arms together as if to clap. On recovery, you can either power back or use an easy breaststroke pull to return to the start. For back butterflies, pull arms back to the starting position with the back of the hand leading.

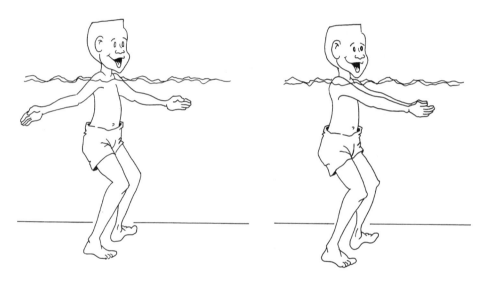

CURL

Objective
Muscular endurance in the upper arm (biceps, power phase up or forward; triceps, power phase down or back)

Description
Stand in a stride position. Extend arms to your side, palms facing forward. Pull the water up, bending the elbow (flexion). If you lengthen your stride to lean forward a little and start with the arms extended behind the body, you can pull forward and then up and get more resistance. For triceps, press down and back to return to the starting position.

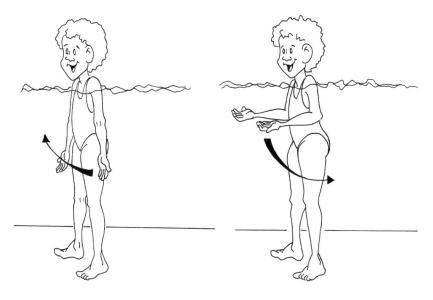

Variations

- Turn palms down.
- Alternate arms in opposition.
- Use a kickboard for triceps curls. Place the board on the surface of the water next to your body. Place your hands in the middle of the board and extend the arm to your side, pressing the board down.

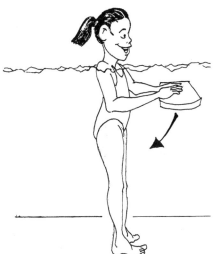

POOL PUSH-UP

Objectives
Strength and muscular endurance in the latissimus dorsi and triceps

Description
Face the wall and place the hands about shoulder-width apart on the deck. Without jumping to get momentum, press yourself up and out of the water using

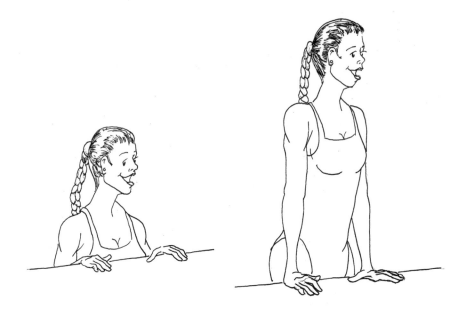

only your arms. Relax and drop back down into the water. For more challenge, bend the knees so that the feet are not touching the bottom of the pool when you begin. You can also do these in the deep water at the wall.

PULL-DOWN

Objective
Muscular endurance in the latissimus dorsi, lower chest fibers, and abdominals

Description
Extend arms out to the side (shoulder abduction), palms down. Pull arms down to the sides. Return to the starting position.

Variations

- Pull down in front of the body.
- Pull down behind the back.
- Pull one hand down in front and the other in back at the same time.

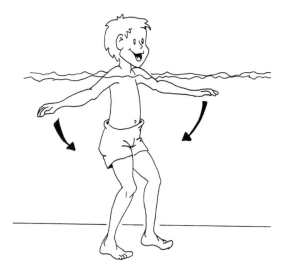

- Alternate front and back pull-downs.
- Pull down with a noodle (using all variations).
- Pull down in front of the body using a kickboard.

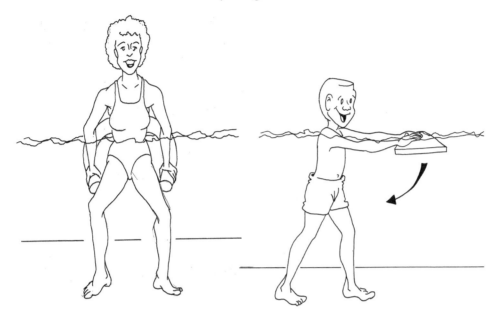

LATERAL RAISE

Objective
Muscular endurance in the upper shoulder muscles (deltoids)

Description
Stand in a straddle position with arms at your sides and palms facing the body. Pull arms laterally away from the body (shoulder abduction). Return to the start position.

Variation
Work Around the Clock: Pull forward and up to midnight (shoulder flexion) and return to the start. Continue pulling up with arms in 11-1 position, 10-2 position, and 9-3 position (shoulder abduction as described previously).

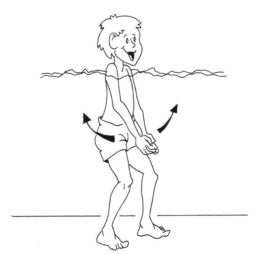

FIGURE EIGHT (SCULLING)

Objective
Muscular endurance in the shoulder girdle muscles, pectoralis, and triceps

Description
Bend the arms in front of the chest and draw figure eights across and just under the surface of the water with your forearms. (Pretend to smooth sand or conduct an orchestra.)

   This exercise is a lead-up skill for more advanced swimming stunts. See chapter 6 for more details on using sculling for support, changing position, and advanced swimming skills.

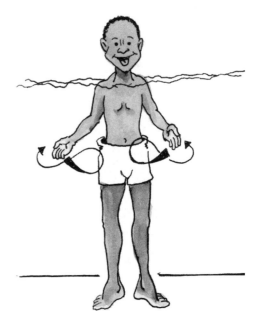

KICKBOARD ROWING

Objective
Muscular endurance in the trapezius, latissimus dorsi, and core muscles, especially the abdominal obliques

Equipment
One kickboard per participant

Description
Hold a kickboard on the sides with both hands. Reach the board out in front and slightly to one side of the body. Dig the bottom edge of the board into the water and paddle back. Recover the board out of the water to the starting position.

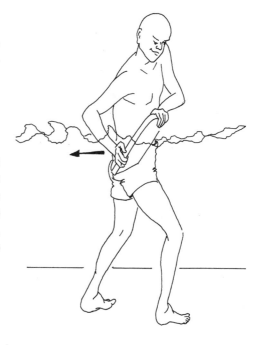

Aqua Basics

The aqua basics described here are variations of jogging, lunges, kicks, and jumping jacks. These moves can all be done with a single-leg variation; in other words, plant one foot on the bottom and go through half of the move with the other leg. Sometimes this is less intense than alternating the motions, but in some cases it is actually harder to do (when speed is held constant). Most of the basics can also be performed at different levels: bouncing, neutral, rebounding, and suspended.

- *Bouncing* refers to bouncing up and down off the toes and lifting the feet off the bottom between steps. Bouncing in slow motion creates a float phase that can be used as an active rest between interval sets. Jogging, hopping, and skipping in slow motion are appropriate for warm-up, cool-down, and recovery segments of interval sets.

- *Neutral* means staying at one level. The core (torso) is held tight and does not change levels, and the shoulders do not noticeably go up and down out of the water. Position yourself as if sitting at the edge of an imaginary high stool. The goal is to work through the water instead of floating through the work. Neutral activities are safer than rebounding because there is not as much impact on the joints during landing. Neutral exercise is recommended for anyone with joint problems.

- *Rebounding* is a variation of bouncing executed with power. Bounce powerfully off the bottom of the pool and try to get more height from step to step. Rebounding is fun and intense if done forcefully with speed. It involves impact on the bottom of the pool that puts stress on the joints. It is appropriate for sport aqua because land athletes often perform powerful jumps, leaps, and rebounds. You will need to limit rebounding if participants complain of pain in their ankles, knees, hips, or lower backs.

- *Suspended* moves are ones in which arm power is used to keep the feet off the bottom of the pool. For most of us it is very intense because with suspended moves we don't use the bottom to help change directions and the arms work overtime to keep us from touching the bottom. Suspending a move is a lead-up for treading water and is a great confidence builder.

Once you have tried all of the basics in these four positions to determine their relative intensities at different speeds, you can begin to add a *travel* variation. Try to move each of the basics across the pool, moving forward, to the side, and backward.

The building blocks include variations in a progression of increasing intensity. You can use the progressions to develop a program and individual workouts. To design a program, determine the fitness goals of the program and the length of the program, and then gradually, over a period of workouts, add intensity by using the progressive sequence described here.

When designing the workout, build from easier (warm-up) to more intense (aerobics or aerobic intervals) exercise using the following sequence. Reverse the progressions to return to easier exercise and begin a cool-down.

Progressive Sequence

- Work in place, easy bouncing, neutral, suspended
- Travel, easy bouncing, then work in place doing a set of repetitions of a predetermined skill or set of skills
- Travel back and repeat the set of repetitions
- Travel forward, turn and travel back, then stop in place, and do a set of repetitions of a predetermined skill or set of skills
- Travel continuously, no break
- Repeat the travel sequence using the neutral position
- Repeat with suspended travel
- Repeat the suspended travel sequence and, when working in place, use rebounding to repeat the skill set

If participants can travel while suspended, they have learned to tread water and to swim without putting their faces in, and they are doing the most intense work in the progressive sequence.

Be sure to observe standard safety precautions for exercise safety when you ask participants to perform any of the activities in this book. These include but are not limited to the following:

- Always perform a good warm-up before increasing the intensity of any of the exercises.
- Try to perform exercises through your entire functional range of motion.
- Do not lock the knees or elbows in the performance of the exercise.
- Do not perform an exercise in which the arms transition from a position under the water to a position above the water.
- Do not hyperextend the lower back or cervical spine with momentum.
- Do not combine flexion or extension of the spine with rotation.
- Try not to exercise entirely on the balls of your feet.
- Always include a cool-down and stretch following your workout.
- If it hurts, don't do it.

MARCHING AND JOGGING

Objectives
Muscular endurance in the back leg muscles (hamstrings and gastrocnemius); cardiorespiratory endurance; interval training

Description
March as on land. Lift one knee up to hip height and then push the foot back to the bottom, then repeat with the other knee. There should always be one foot in contact with the bottom (that is, no float phase).

Jog as on land. In the neutral position, pretend to sit on a high stool and jog without bouncing up and down. There is a float phase in this skill. You will discover that if speed and range of motion are the same, the march is more intense than the jog.

Variations and Progressions
Jog or march depending on how hard you want to work.

- Jog forward with breaststroke.
- Jog backward with chest butterflies.
- Jog forward with chest butterflies.
- Jog backward with breaststroke.
- Jog forward with biceps curls.
- Jog backward with triceps curls.

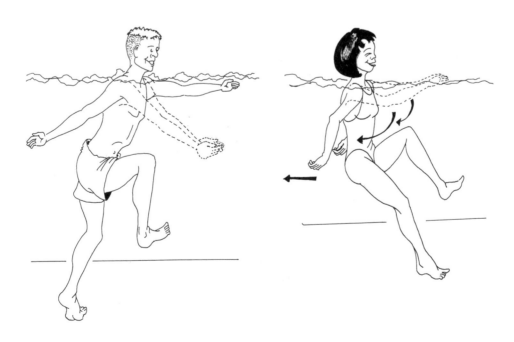

MOUNTAIN CLIMBER

Objectives
Stretching; muscular endurance in upper leg muscles (hamstrings, glutei); cardio-respiratory endurance

Description
Begin in a stride position. Bend the knee of the rear leg and bring it forward to a position hip high (as if getting ready to climb stairs, three steps at a time). Return to the stride (like a rear lunge). Repeat with the same leg. Repeat the motion on the other side. (Because this move is designed to have one foot in contact with the floor, suspended position is not applicable.)

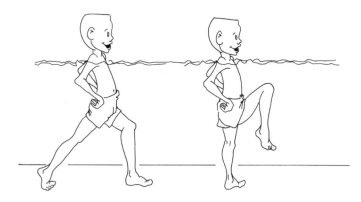

KICKER

Objectives
Muscular endurance and flexibility in the muscles of the upper leg (quadriceps, hip flexors, hamstrings, and glutei); cardiorespiratory endurance

Description
Begin by standing erect, with legs together and the hands by the sides. Lift the legs, one at a time, (with knee slightly bent) toward the surface of the water. Start low and then kick up higher. Do not kick higher than hip level. Use opposing rhythm with the arms (such as curls or, to challenge coordination, try the crawlstroke or pull-downs). Kicking can be performed with a float phase, which makes it easier, or as a march, in which one foot returns to the bottom before the other leg begins the next kick.

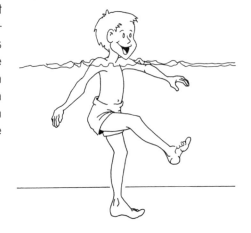

Variations

- *Vertical flutter kick:* Knees and ankles remain relaxed. Kick just off the bottom of the pool as if trying to kick your shoes across the room.
- *Soccer kick:* Pretend to kick a soccer ball up to yourself.
- *Kick Around the Clock:* Using neutral or rebound, alternate leg kicks to the following positions on the face of an imaginary clock; kick right and left toward 12, kick right to 1 and left to 11, kick right to 2 and left to 10, and then repeat as desired.
- For kicking with equipment, see Independent Kicking in chapter 6 (page 125).
- *Russian kicks:* Squat slightly on an imaginary stool (neutral position) and kick the legs one at a time, extending the lower leg to a 45-degree straddle position.

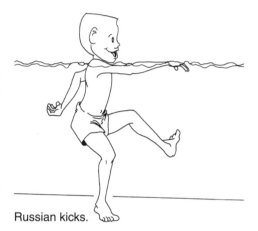

Russian kicks.

SCISSORS

Objectives

Stretching; muscular endurance in the glutei (lead-up for Cross-Country Ski, page 46); cardiorespiratory endurance

Description

From the standing position with legs together, lunge backward on one leg as the other leg lunges forward into a stride position. Move legs in a scissors-like motion and repeat. Work arms in opposition. You can use shoulder flexion (raise the arm forward and up from the shoulder joint), biceps curls, or lateral raises with the elbows bent.

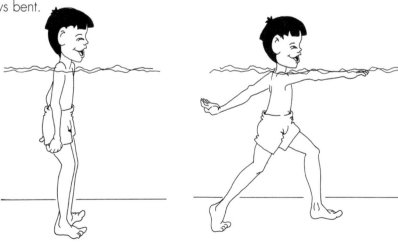

Variation
Countdowns: Begin with 10 scissors, right leg in front. Follow with 10 scissors, left leg in front. Then continue to count down, 9 scissors, 8 scissors, and so on.

CROSS-COUNTRY SKI

Objectives
Stretching; muscular endurance in the hip flexors and extensors and glutei; cardio-respiratory endurance

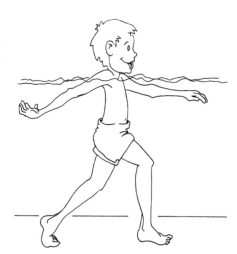

Description
Begin in a stride position. Switch strides. Work arms in opposition (shoulder flexion and extension). For less effort on the shoulders, slice the hands through the water; for more effort, turn the palms down throughout the shoulder work to create resistance for the anterior and posterior deltoids.

Variations
- *Stride wide:* Same as previously, but straddle the legs about shoulder-width apart. Swing the arms side to side in front of the body.
- *Ski walk:* Shorten the steps, pump the arms as if running, and travel forward or backward.

BUTT KICKER

Objectives
Stretching; warm-up

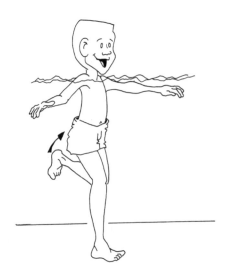

Description
Begin by standing erect, with legs together and the arms by the side. Pull the heel of one foot toward the butt, keeping the knee directly under the hip. Do one leg at a time (singles) or alternate legs.

Safety
Be sure to stabilize the torso to keep from hyperextending the back. Do not perform this for intervals or cardiorespiratory endurance.

JUMPING JACK

Objectives

Muscular endurance in the abductors and adductors of hips and shoulders; warm-up or cool-down; muscle isolation

Description

Begin by standing erect, with the legs together and the arms by the side with palms facing the legs. Abduct shoulders and hips and then return to the starting position. Keep the arms below the surface of the water to take advantage of the water resistance.

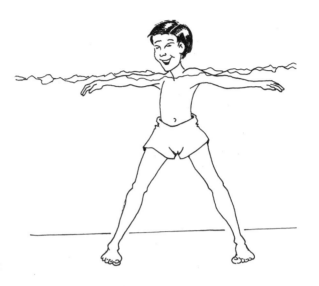

Variations

- *Side lunge:* Start as stated previously but step out to the side with one foot and return. Repeat on the same side, or alternate sides. Use the lateral raise.

- *Step side:* Step to the side as a side lunge and continue moving in that direction as you bring the trail leg to the lead leg. Use the lateral raise or challenge with curls.   .

- *Jack crossover:* Do the standard jumping jack but instead of stopping with the legs together, cross the legs and arms right over left or vice-versa.

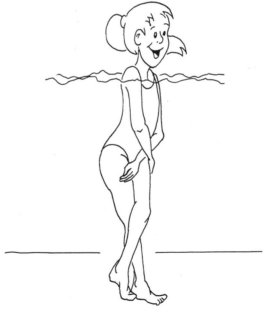

Jack crossover.

- *Limbo jack:* From a standing position, with the hands on the hips or about head high out of the water, perform the leg crossovers described in jack crossover. Progressively bend the knees more and more during the crossover jacks to "see how low you can go," and then return to standing height.
- *Jack shuffle:* Travel sideways across the pool using the jack crossover.

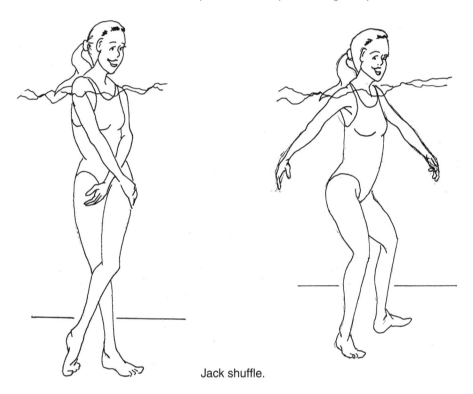

Jack shuffle.

- *Pop-up:* To work the adductor muscles, start in a straddle position (hips abducted) and pop up off the bottom pulling the legs together as your feet leave the bottom. Do not lock the knees and do not move explosively with speed or power, or you could hurt the adductor muscles of the inner thigh.
- *Noodle jacks:* Grab the ends of a noodle and perform pop-ups as previously described. Pull the noodle down behind you to work the latissimus dorsi.

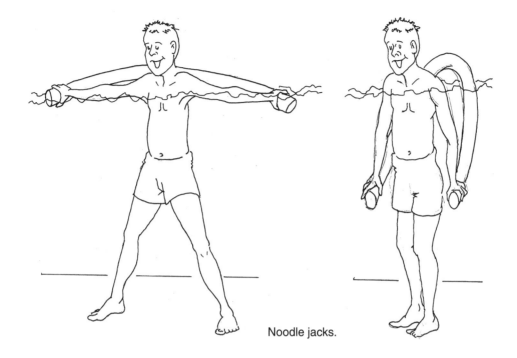
Noodle jacks.

Sport Aqua

Water workouts are excellent for sport training and conditioning and are much easier on the joints than land exercise. Basketball and volleyball players, cheerleaders, tennis players, and runners can all rebound in jumps, kicks, and jacks and still have softer landings than during land training. In preseason, water workouts provide resistance to movement to help develop muscular endurance. During the season, incorporating sport aqua into the regular practice schedule keeps athletes fresh and helps reduce muscle soreness. In addition, water slows movement, and buoyancy and hydrostatic pressure support balance, making it easier to practice techniques (such as kickboxing) in slow motion.

Sport aqua activities can also be used effectively for any age group to increase challenge and interject more variety into the workout. The only additional precaution that should be observed is that with populations that have balance and coordination issues, you will need to progress slowly through the variations that include quick changes in direction. It is best and safest to stop and work in place before changing direction so that the water turbulence does not affect standing balance.

Remember that water affects movement in unique ways. Not only does the water make you slower, your arms and legs find it easier to follow a path of least resistance. This is why sport aqua skills will not conform exactly to sport-specific biomechanics. However, participants will still experience fun and excitement in the attempt.

Most of the sport aqua skills included in this section are appropriate for any sport that involves running or jumping. You can combine aqua basics with any of the skills listed here to meet a training objective (specifically, cardiorespiratory endurance, aerobic intervals, or anaerobic training). In addition, if you have a teaching or coaching background in a certain sport, you can go to the pool and experiment with ideas to decide if they are appropriate for warm-up, cardiorespiratory endurance, or intervals. The section that follows describes activities that can be used in sport conditioning.

POWER JOG

Objectives
Muscular endurance in the upper legs and anterior and posterior deltoids; interval training; cardiorespiratory endurance

Description
Lean forward and run as hard as you can for a predetermined distance or time. Pump the arms hard as if racing to the tape at the finish line. Keep the knees coming up to hip level. Dropping the knees will reduce the intensity of the power jog.

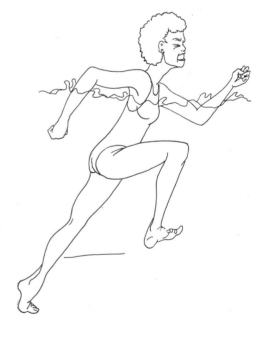

Variations
- *Sprint, pivot, sprint back-ward:* Power jog half of the distance to the boundary. Pivot so that you are facing backward and run the rest of the distance backward. Check that the space behind you is clear before you move backward.

- *Run on the diagonal:* This improves balance, challenges the core muscles, and improves ability to make quick directional changes. Run "on a diagonal" (45-degree angle) for a predetermined number of steps (suggestion: use odd numbers so that the diagonal push is alternated from the right foot to the left foot). After completing the running steps on the diagonal, stop and push off in the opposite direction (again, on the diagonal). For example, run three steps and then push off in the other direction, and continue that pattern.

THREE-STEP JUMP STOP

Objectives
Balance; keeping weight forward on the toes; muscular endurance of the upper legs; cardiorespiratory endurance

Description
Power jog forward for three steps and then jump to a stop with both feet. You will be in a forward semi-squat position with the arms up. If training for basketball, put the hands up in defensive position. Continue three-step jump stop for a predetermined distance.

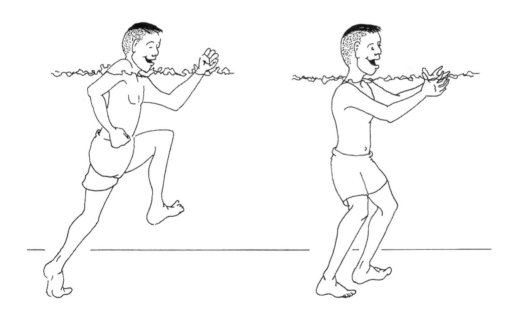

Variation
After completing the jump stop, complete a predetermined number of vertical jumps with the hands reaching up, as in a rebound.

DEFENSIVE SLIDE

Objectives
Muscular endurance of the adductors and abductors of the thigh; footwork and balance; cardiorespiratory endurance

Description
Position the hands as if to catch a pass, or in defensive position for basketball. Bend the knees slightly and slide sideways to travel a predetermined distance.

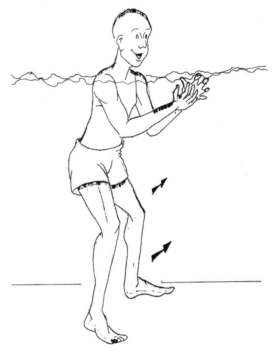

Variations
- *Partner ball pass:* Using any type of activity ball, perform the defensive slide facing a partner and pass the ball back and forth between you. This will improve eye–hand coordination and ball-handling skill.

- To improve the muscular power of the upper body, give each person a kickboard and perform a chest pass (do not release the board but perform only the passing motion with the kickboard) as you slide. You can do this either as an individual or a partner activity.

- Combine the defensive slide with a rebound vertical jump.

- *Four Corners:* Slide across the pool, backpedal for a short distance, slide back the other direction, then power jog forward. This formation looks like a square. Add a rebound at each corner. To overload progressively, on round one perform one jump, on round two perform two jumps, and so on. Don't forget to reverse direction to work on the muscles of the other leg. Muscular balance is the key to staying injury free.

TIRE RUN

Objectives
Muscular endurance in the hip abductors and hamstrings; balance; leg power; cardiorespiratory endurance

Description
Jog with the legs in a straddle position. Pull the knees up high and jog forward as if to maneuver through a set of imaginary football tires.

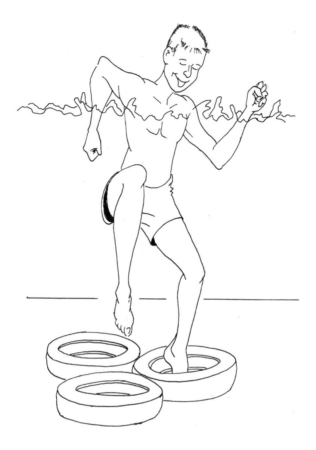

GRAPEVINE

Objectives
Balance; muscular endurance of the abductors and adductors of the thigh; foot speed; cardiorespiratory endurance

Description
Travel to the side, crossing the right foot over the left foot. Step sideways with the left and then cross the right foot behind the left foot. Continue traveling sideways,

alternating cross in front, cross behind. After a predetermined distance, reverse the steps to move the other direction. Use your arms to move the water to help with balance and propulsion, or hold them in front of the body or in defensive position.

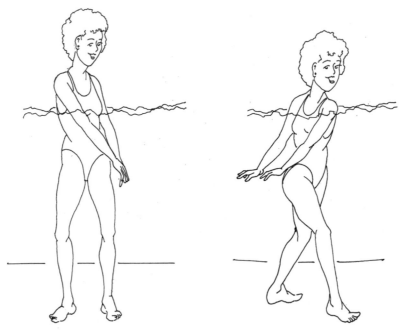

HILL TOPPER

Objectives
Muscular endurance in the upper legs; flexibility in the hips, knees, ankles, and feet; cardiorespiratory endurance; interval training

Description
Face the wall and position yourself about an arm's width away. Pretend to sprint up the wall (the hill), putting one foot up the wall ahead of the other and pumping the arms in opposition to assist the upward

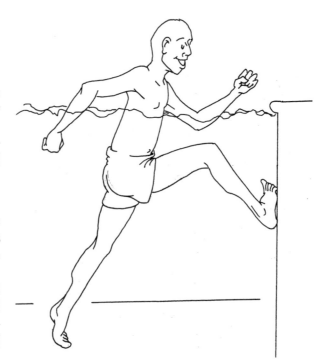

climb. As you try to climb the hill, make sure that your foot contacts the wall on the ball of your foot and keep the ankle flexed.

POWER KNEE LIFT

Objectives
Quick feet; muscular endurance in the upper legs; cardiorespiratory endurance; interval training

Description
Partners stand facing each other. One person extends her hands toward her partner, just under the surface of the water, to offer a target. The partner performs a predetermined number (or a time limit, for intervals) of power knee lifts, trying to touch her knees to the palms of her partner's hands (hit the target). Change roles and repeat. Power knee lifts are done much too fast to attempt other arm variations.

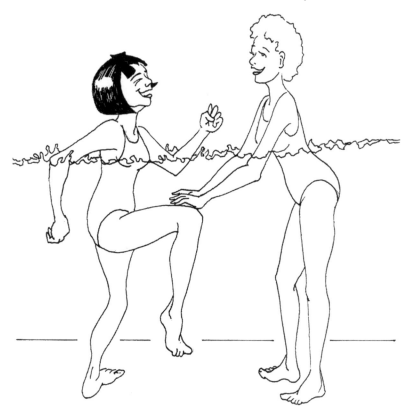

Variation
Have the partner holding the hands out shuffle backward in a short ski-walk motion while the other person tries to knee-lift forward and hit the target. The partner should check that the space is clear before moving backward.

ROPE JUMP

Objectives
Stretching; muscular endurance in quadriceps, hamstrings, and gastrocnemius (calf muscle); cardiorespiratory endurance

Description
Pretend to jump rope (hop on both feet). Arms remain underwater with the upper arms pressed to the side. Swing a pretend rope overhead forward or backward. Combine with kickboxing basics to plan a workout (see sample at the end of the chapter). If you have experience in kickboxing, use your imagination to add to or vary the use of the imaginary jump rope in your workout.

Variations
- *Jog:* Jog while turning the rope and travel forward, backward, or to either side.
- *Hop on one foot:* Add a moderate level of impact and work on dynamic balance by hopping on one foot. Pull the heel of the other foot back gently or hold at 90-degree hip flexion.
- *Razzle Dazzle:* For extra endurance of shoulders and triceps, try making figure eights with the rope as you jog.
- *Skip:* Pretend to skip the rope. Alternate a right knee lift with a left butt kicker, then jog the rope to make the transition to the other side (left knee lift with a right butt kicker).

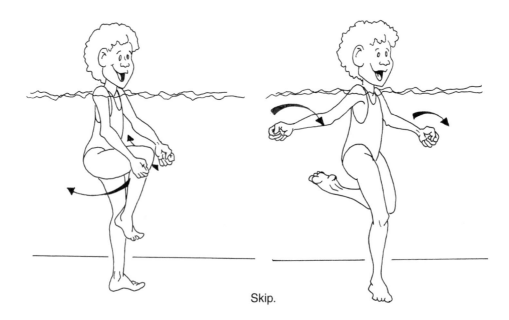

Skip.

SKIP BOUNDING

Objectives
Leg and arm strength and power; muscular endurance in the quadriceps, hamstrings, and glutei; interval training

Description
Skip forward, bounding up off the bottom with each new step. Work the arms in opposition: one is driving forward and up to the surface of the water and the other is pressing down and back to balance the skipping motion.

Safety
In shallow water, participants may pull the arms forcefully out of the water. Encourage them to decelerate to keep the arms from breaking the water. Moving with momentum from water resistance to air resistance can injure the shoulder muscles.

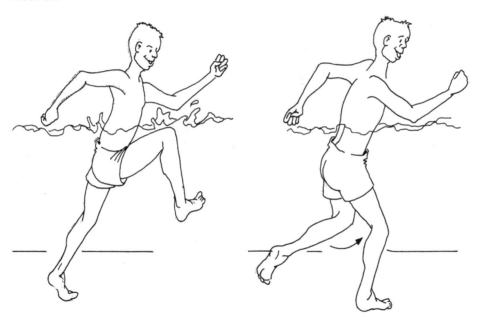

CHEST PASS

Objective
Muscular endurance in the pectoralis group, anterior deltoids, and triceps

Equipment
One kickboard per participant

Description

Use a kickboard to simulate a ball and to increase the resistance of the skill. Hold the board perpendicular to the water and grip the side edges. Pull the board just under the surface of the water and push the board away from you as if passing a basketball to a partner. If you pull the board back into your chest forcefully, you will improve muscular balance by working the upper-back muscles and the posterior deltoids.

Variations

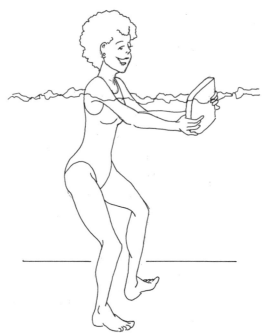

- *Partner chest pass:* Perform the skill facing a partner to increase the water pressure.

- *Chest pass with rotation:* To work the abdominal obliques, rotate the torso right to press the board to the right. Bring it back to center and then repeat to the left side, always bringing the board back to a position next to the chest before rotating to the other side.

THREE-PERSON WEAVE

Objectives

Eye–hand coordination; muscular endurance of the legs; cardiorespiratory endurance

Equipment

An activity ball approximately the same size as a basketball or volleyball

Description

Working in groups of three, start with participants standing next to each other in a line on a boundary. The person in the middle has the ball. As the group begins to jog forward, the person in the middle passes to the person on the right and follows the pass, moving behind the participant receiving the pass. The participant with the ball passes to the other player and then weaves behind her. The three continue to weave forward to the next boundary. The key to this drill is to move behind the player you pass to and continue to the other side of the group to receive each successive pass. If viewed from above, it would look like a figure eight pattern.

Variation

Use a progression of intensity and ball skills challenges by starting the group out standing close together. Gradually increase the distance between the players. The farther apart they are, the harder they have to work in the water to cover the required distance.

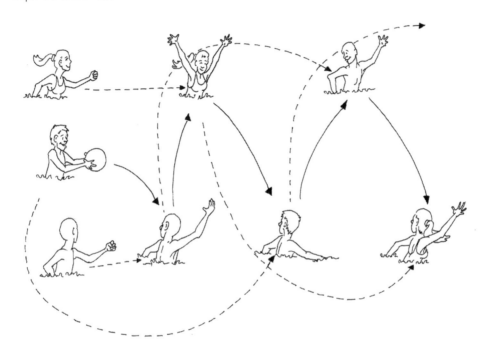

REBOUND

Objectives

Vertical jump (a measure of leg power); muscular endurance in the hamstrings, quadriceps, and glutei; interval training

Description

Start with the legs shoulder-width apart and hands held about head high. Bend the knees to squat until the water is at your chin (loading the hips) and jump up as high as you can, reaching the arms overhead as if to block a volleyball spike or rebound a basketball.

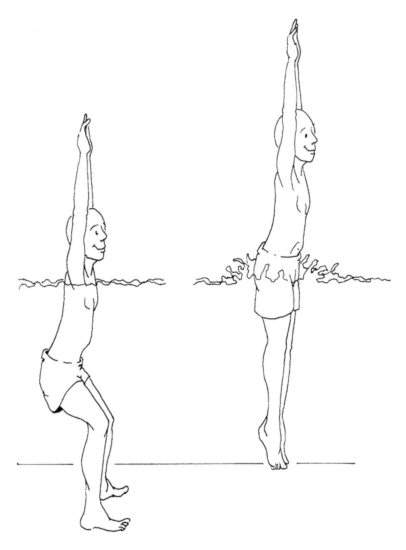

Variations

- *Partner blocks:* Face a partner. As you jump, try to clap hands with your partner at the top of the block.

- *Jump and spin:* Do partner blocks, but try to spin one full rotation after your feet leave the bottom before clapping hands with your partner.

- *Hitch kicks:* To overload the hamstrings, perform blocks and partner blocks; as you jump, pull the heels up toward the buttocks. Be careful not to hyperextend the back.

SKI JUMP

Objective
Muscular endurance in the abdominal muscles, in particular the obliques in lateral flexion (bending to the side)

Description
Begin with legs together. Lift both feet off the bottom by flexing the knees forward. Land to the right of center. Lift the feet again and land to the left of center. Use the arms to pull the water in opposition to the leg lifts. The motion is similar to the action of a person parallel skiing down a mountain.

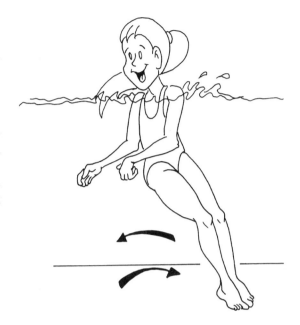

Kickboxing Basics

Kickboxing has become a very popular form of aerobic activity in recent years and has been introduced in the water. However, kickboxing basics must be modified from land aerobics or competitive applications because the water slows movement and changes the biomechanics. Kickboxing basics for the water are designed for group fitness application and not for competition. The kicks and punches are similar to those on land, but you will need to modify the footwork (combinations of traveling, kicks, and punches) because water slows you down too much for land applications to be as effective. Other modifications include providing more room for the participants to kick and punch without contacting other participants and modifying applications that use music for choreography or motivation. If you have training in kickboxing you can use your knowledge to add to the ideas in this section of the chapter.

Before beginning this section we will describe the starting positions for these skills. There are two variations of the boxer's stance. Always start facing your target. You have the option of positioning the feet either in a straddle or with one foot staggered back. Buoyancy will help you keep the weight on the balls of the feet. Keep the arms close to the body, protecting the head and the heart. Maintain an erect posture. Keep the core tight, the shoulders back and down, and the ribcage lifted. Kicks and punches are executed with two concentric phases (the muscle shortens to create movement). The water helps decelerate the kick or punch to keep the limbs from overextending.

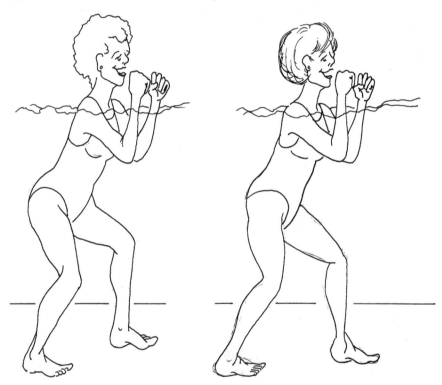

PUNCHES

Objective
Muscular endurance for pectoralis, triceps, and deltoids

Description
Stand in a boxer's stance and punch as described:

> *Jab:* Punch forward and pronate the arm (turn it so the palm faces down) as you extend the arm at the elbow to deliver the punch. Retract to the start

position. Target the head of an imaginary opponent. If you stand in a straddle position you will be able to punch with either arm and rotate the trunk toward the target. In a staggered stance, punch only with the lead arm.

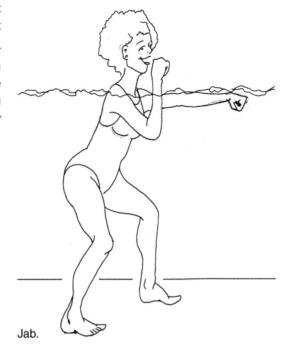

Jab.

Cross: Punch as in the jab, but cross over the midline of the body. From a staggered stance, rotate the torso and pivot on the back foot to create a straight line into the punch. Retract arm to boxer's stance position.

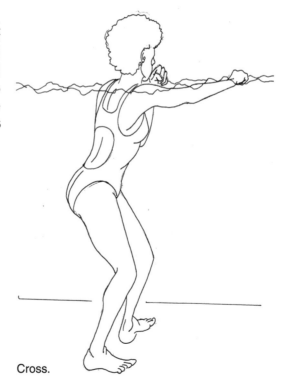

Cross.

Hook: This punch is thrown in a circular motion, with the target being the opponent's cheek (side of the face). Abduct the arm at the shoulder (lateral raise) keeping the elbow bent. Rotate the trunk as you punch with a hooking action toward the midline of the body. Retract the arm back to the rib cage.

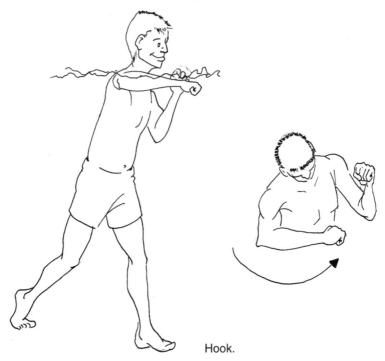

Hook.

Uppercut: Use a staggered stance to start this punch with a windup. Circle the arm to bring the elbow past the rib cage to a position behind you. Then, targeting the opponent's ribs or chin, throw the punch away from your body. The lower body essentially lunges into the punch and the abdominal muscles contract to pull the pelvis forward into the punch. The back foot pivots into the punch.

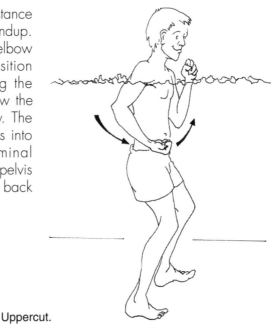

Uppercut.

FRONT KICK

Objectives
Dynamic balance; muscular endurance in the quadriceps and hamstrings

Description
Assume a boxer's stance. Contract the core muscles. Execute hip flexion first and follow with leg extension to contact an imaginary opponent at the knee, shin, or torso. The leg will be extended in front of you at the height of your imaginary target, and the foot is flexed to contact the target with the ball of the foot. Quickly flex the knee and then return to the boxer's stance. Kick height depends on strength, flexibility, and balance. Higher kicks are more difficult.

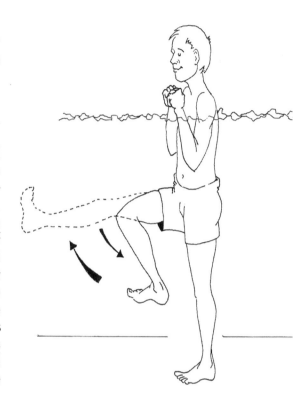

SIDE KICK

Objectives
Dynamic balance; muscular endurance in the hamstrings, glutei (especially the gluteus medius), and hip abductors

Description
Use a straddle stance. Contract the core muscles. Start by abducting the hip with the knee bent to bring the foot to the height of the imaginary target (knee or lower torso). Keep the hip, knee, and toes pointing forward toward the target. Extend the leg at the knee, contacting the target with the top of the foot. Quickly flex the knee and then return to the boxer's stance. Kick height depends on strength, flexibility, and balance, although you should not try to kick the foot out of the water.

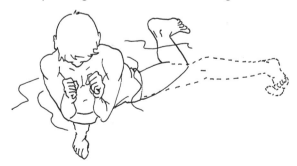

Workout Design

In this section we will discuss various formations for the workouts. The type of workout that you design using aqua basics and sport aqua depends on the age and interest of the participants. However, we have tried these same activities with all age groups and regardless of age most participants enjoy the comfort and support of the water and the challenge of the activity. They also enjoy formations that get them working with a partner or in a game activity, and often we find them to be highly competitive with the sport aqua skills.

There are a number of ways to organize the basics for effectiveness and fun. These include circles, line formations, and circuits.

Circles

Circles are fun and social and get the water moving to increase the difficulty of the skills. For less resistance, continue in the same direction for the entire set. The water begins to push you around and assist movement (because of inertia). For more resistance, change direction frequently and you will have to work hard just to keep moving around the circle.

Circles work well in pools that slope gently toward deeper water. In pools with quick changes in depths, shorter participants will struggle to make forward progress when they reach deeper water.

Moving water can sweep an unsuspecting participant off his feet. Keep a close eye on participants who seem apprehensive about the movement of the water and be sure there is a safety rope in place dividing the shallow water from the deep (shallow is 5 feet [about 1.5 meters] or less). Here is a sample circle workout.

SAMPLE CIRCLE WORKOUT

This is known as the **big circle–little circle** format. Organize participants in a circle standing shoulder to shoulder facing the inside of the circle. Ask them to take a giant step back and do a jumping jack to make sure there is enough room to move. This determines the size of the little circle (LC). The size of the big circle (BC) is determined by the size of the playing area. Have all participants back the circle up to the boundaries of the playing area. This is how big the BC should be during the activity.

The intent of the circle format is to move participants in all directions including clockwise (CW) and counterclockwise (CCW) around the circle. For example, facing the circle and jogging backward using butterflies makes the circle bigger (BC), and jogging forward with breaststroke makes the circle smaller (LC). You can also turn your back to the center of the circle and travel forward and back.

Turning the right shoulder toward the center of the circle and traveling forward is clockwise. Turning the left shoulder toward the center of the circle and moving forward is counterclockwise. With the right shoulder in the center of the circle stepping to the side, moving left makes the circle bigger and vice versa. As you practice the sample workout, don't worry if everyone misses a cue and moves differently than the others—just keep everyone moving.

Variations

- *Circle within a circle:* Make the circles go in opposite directions so that participants create turbulence for each other.
- Use a Follow the Leader approach with the big circle–little circle format. Each person directs the group from a big circle to a little circle, goes around once, and then moves back to the big circle. Follow the Leader is described on page 94.

Key

From

    LC Little circle
    BC Big circle

Facing

    F Forward
    RS Right shoulder in
    LS Left shoulder in
    B Backward

Moving with the activity

    In place
    Move forward
    Move backward
    Move CW
    Move CCW
    Move right
    Move left

Start in the little circle formation.

From	Facing	Moving with the activity
LC	F	March in place
LC	F	March—move backward with butterflies
BC	F	March in place
BC	RS	March—move CW with breaststroke
BC	RS	Step side—move right to LC
LC	RS	Step side—move left to BC
BC	LS	Jog—move CCW with breaststroke
BC	LS	Jog backward—move CW with butterflies
BC	F	Ski in place

(continued)

(continued)

From	Facing	Moving with the activity
BC	F	Ski—move forward
LC	F	Butt kickers—in place—with sculling (figure eights)
LC	F	Butt kickers—move backward with butterflies
BC	F	Jumping jacks in place
BC	RS	2 steps—move right to LC 2 steps—move left to BC—repeat 4 times
BC	LS	Jog—move CCW about 20 steps Turn to right—move CW Repeat 4 times
BC	F	Ski—move forward to LC Ski—move backward to BC
BC	F	Jumping jacks—quarter-turn with each jack until you have completed 1 turn, then reverse the turn
BC	RS	2 steps—move right to LC 2 steps—move left to BC—side kicks with the left leg Repeat from 2 steps—move right 4 times
BC	F	Jog 3 steps and front kick in place Repeat 8 times
BC	F	Jog—move forward Ski—move back
BC	F	Repeat workout from the top

You can do this workout all of the way through in slow motion to warm up and then gradually add speed to increase resistance and effort for the cardiorespiratory endurance set.

Line Formations

Line formations are a great way to begin partner work. Partners face each other and move toward and away from each other as they progress through the workout. Pair people who are of similar size, weight, and strength, especially if they will hook elbows or push and pull each other through a skill. Here are some sample workouts that use line formations.

SAMPLE LINE WORKOUT 1

Form two lines 6 to 10 feet apart. Have partners face each other, then move forward toward their partners (address the partners) to begin the workout. Perform the skills and then move back to the original line. You need to select the locomotor move to be used to travel forward and back when addressing the partner. Begin slowly for warm-up and then increase the speed a little at a time. To use this formation for interval training, perform the activities one after another without returning to the starting point in line. Then on the rest interval, change activities or start the line process over slowly with new skills.

- Travel to your partner and back to the line using jogging with breast-stroke
- Link right elbows and swing your partner
- Trade places in the line with jogging and breaststroke
- Link left elbows and swing your partner
- Trade places in the line with jogging and breaststroke
- 10 power knee lifts each
- Trade places in the line with jogging and breaststroke
- 10 rebounds
- Trade places in the line with jogging and breaststroke
- 10 pop-up jacks

SAMPLE LINE WORKOUT 2

Start out slowly with a warm-up and speed up the activities to create intervals. Form two lines 6 to 10 feet apart. Partners face each other.

- Jog forward, clap hands with your partner, butt kicker back. Use breaststroke or crawlstroke arm actions to travel forward and reverse breaststroke to travel backward.
- Jog forward, clap your hands, butt kicker back.
- Jog forward, link elbows with partner. Swing your partner right, then left.
- Jog back to the line.

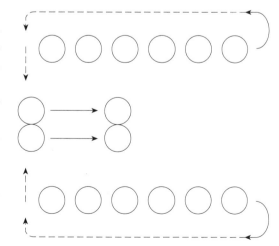

- Do-si-do by crossing your arms over your chest and passing shoulders with your partner. Return to the line.
- Promenade by jogging to the center, meeting your partner, and marching down the line. One couple goes at a time. As soon as the first couple is halfway down the line, the next set of partners promenades. The promenade line continues until everyone has returned to the starting position. Promenade using different exercises described in the previous section (such as jogging, kicks, jacks, tire jog, ski shuffle, jack shuffle, fancy footwork, and so on).
- Join hands, circle right 10 steps, circle left 10 steps.
- Swing your partner right, then left.
- Return to line formation.

Variation *The Grand March:* Each person chooses a partner, and all partners form two lines about 6 feet apart (participants stand one behind the other and face forward). The dance begins with the partners at the back of the lines jogging forward between the two lines. As they reach the head of the line, they turn right and jog back on the outside of the line. Each successive pair jogs down the middle of the lines, and every other group turns right and the others go left. When they reach the back of the line the two partners on the right pair with the partners on the left and go down the middle of the lines as a group of four. Continue this process until there are groups of eight. The eights then make a circle. Continue with the selected activities in the circles. Try letting the groups do a Follow the Leader format where each participant picks a new skill, moving to a new leader around the circle until everyone has had a turn.

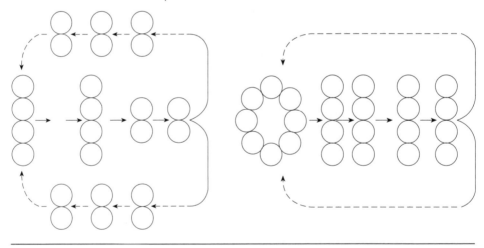

Aqua Circuit

The aqua circuit is designed to improve cardiorespiratory endurance and muscular endurance using only the water for the resistance. It is also an opportunity for participants to work at their own pace, by themselves or with a partner, to accomplish the training goal of the day. Be sure that you have taught all of the sport aqua skills, arm works, or aqua basics that you will include in the circuit. Provide a group warm-up before beginning the circuit.

To plan your circuit, you will need to do the following:

• *Determine the number of stations needed.* Make an activity card and tape it to an orange traffic cone (pylon) at each station. Walk the participants through the circuit and demonstrate the activity at each station. Before participants begin, decide on a start and stop signal.

• *Determine the amount of time or the number of repetitions to be completed at each station.* To keep participants on task you can play music with a heavy, constant beat and ask them to do the exercise to the beat. Music from 100 to 120 beats per minute will work well if you want to stay on beat. You can use 125 to 140 if you exercise on the half-beat (move to every other beat instead of every beat).

If you want cardiorespiratory endurance to be one of the goals, have participants exercise with 70 percent effort and then jog to the next station. Go around the circuit a predetermined number of times (recommended three sets). For example, review the following:

Circuit time for three rotations: 30 minutes

Total elapsed time with warm-up and cool-down: 50 minutes

Begin together as a group. Warm up (10 minutes) by doing jogging, kickers, cross-country ski, butt kickers, and jumping jacks. Then divide the group equally among the stations.

Perform 30 to 45 seconds of exercise at each station. Change stations by jogging to the new station. Perform three rotations of the circuit.

Sample Workout

Butterflies

Rebound

Pull-down (emphasize the pull-down, relax to starting position)

Power knee lifts

Kickboard rowing

Hill toppers

Curls (emphasize the pull-up, relax and return to the start position for biceps)

Side kicks

Curls (emphasize the press-down, relax for triceps)

Front kicks

Chest press (with the kickboard)

Cool-down and stretch: 10 minutes

chapter 5

Water Games and Relays

Now that you know the basics, you can add water games that train cardiorespiratory and muscular endurance into the workout. Here we will first describe individual and partner stunts and skills that can be incorporated into many of the game formats in this chapter. We'll follow that with relays, tag games, and individual or team events. You will also find variations that include supported swimming skills, in which a partner or equipment aids a participant in maintaining a swimming position without putting his or her face in the water, and variations for participants who know how to swim. There's a sample workout at the end to show you how to put these activities all together for a class.

The games described here are all conducted in shallow water (no more than 5 feet [1.5 meters] deep) so that participants who do not know how to swim or do not swim well can participate fully. To keep game play fair and equal, position shorter participants in shallower water if possible and taller participants in deeper water. Taller participants have a travel advantage, meaning that they can get around faster in shallower water and will gain an advantage in game play if the water is too shallow.

If the game or activity has a swimming variation, you can assume that swimmers have access to the entire pool unless you decide to restrict swimmers to the deep end to reduce a game advantage. This allows you to expand the game and to reduce congestion in shallow water when you are working with a large group. As you plan to incorporate games and activities into your workout, check the Fitness Activity Finder to see if the game is appropriate for warm-up and cool-down phases or for cardiorespiratory endurance or interval training.

Individual and Partner Stunts

Before learning games that train, let's view some brief descriptions of activities that can be used in some of the relays and even in the tag games that follow. We included partner activities in order to meet three main objectives:

• The first is to encourage socialization. Pairing up participants doubles the fun, and if you make certain that participants switch partners frequently, they have the opportunity to get to know everyone within the group.

• The second objective is to provide opportunities for cooperation and problem solving. Participants are often challenged to find a "faster" solution in order to survive a game or successfully complete an activity.

• The third objective is related to the fitness benefit derived from partnering with someone. Partner skills make the water extremely turbulent, which in turn increases the resistance to movement and the challenge to balance so participants will improve their muscular strength. When you incorporate partner skills into the workout or game, those skills contribute to the overall fitness objective.

Observe standard safety precautions (as listed in chapter 3). Partners should be similar in size, strength, and skill unless you pair a weaker person with a stronger person to balance the game play and give everyone similar advantages and disadvantages. Be certain that participants who are comfortable in the water do not inadvertently submerge an unsuspecting participant. If you decide to let participants work with a friend in order to ensure comfort and participation, be sure that the partners are approximately the same size and strength.

PARTNER LOCOMOTION

Objectives
Cardiorespiratory endurance; interval training

Description
One person walks across the pool for a predetermined distance, pushing or pulling, dragging or assisting the partner using the following variations.

- Link elbows facing the same direction and try to travel together using all of the locomotor skills listed in chapter 2.
- Link elbows facing the opposite direction and travel forward, backward, or side to side. Let participants figure out the fastest way to travel under these circumstances.

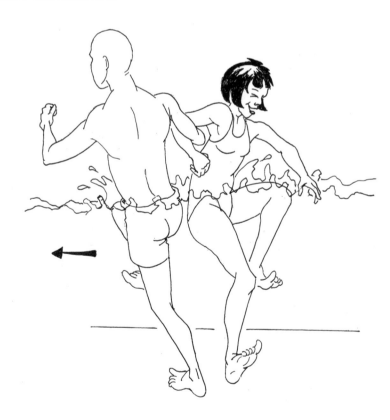

- Partner A begins in a standing position. Partner B grabs partner A at the waist and the two take off to the boundary. While A runs forward, B kicks to assist.

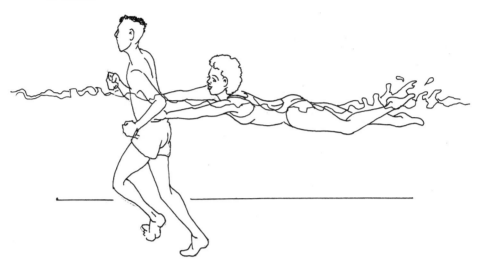

- Partner A begins in a standing position. Partner B is behind on her back and places her feet in the hands of A. Similar to pulling a wheelbarrow, A pulls B across the playing area by the feet. Partner B must keep her face out of the water.

- Begin with groups of three. Two partners link elbows with a third person, who is on his back between them. The partners run forward, pulling the third person with them. The partner being towed tries to remain horizontal to reduce resistance.

When the partners reach a specified boundary, they trade positions and return to the start.

Safety
Make sure all pairs or groups are working in the same direction. Do not let partners hook up by interlacing fingers.

JUMP AND SPIN

Objectives
Vertical jump; body control; interval training

Description
With the arms above the shoulders, jump as high as you can and try to spin around once before your feet touch.

Variation

Partner Jump and Spin: Face your partner and try to jump and spin and clap hands together before your feet touch the bottom. Then try to do a spin and a half. (It's not possible, but it's fun to try!)

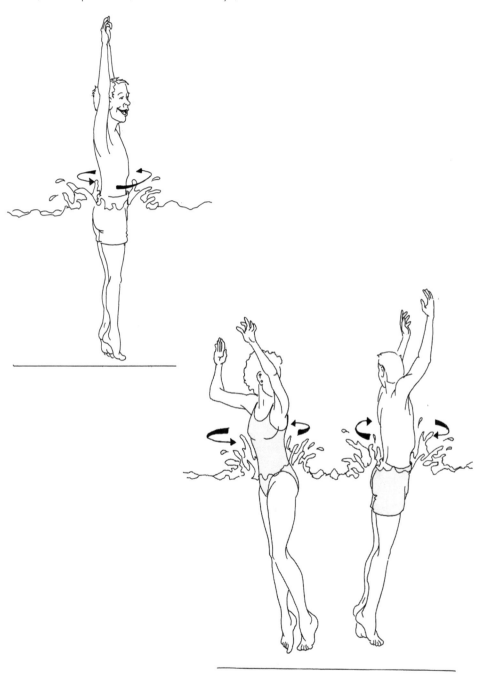

PARTNER JUMP TURN

Objectives
Improve vertical jump; create additional resistance for your partner; change directions in a workout; interval training

Description
Face your partner and grab hands. Jump as high as you can and at the same time try to turn a quarter, half, or full turn before your feet come down.

Safety
Do not interlace fingers.

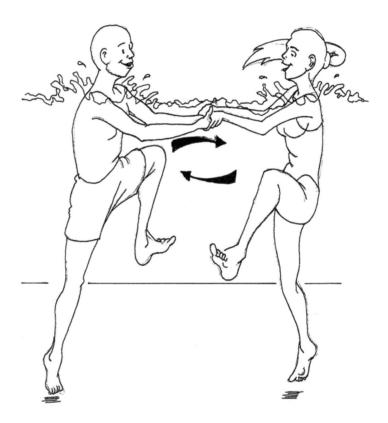

KICKBOARD CRUISING

Objectives
Balance; sculling and stroking skills; muscular endurance

Equipment
One kickboard per participant. If you do not have enough boards, practice these travel skills in a shuttle relay format.

Description

Begin by placing the board behind the knees and balancing in a sitting position. Perform various skills doing the following:

- Use your sculling motion to spin in a circle.

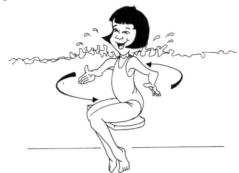

- Row your boat (breaststroke pull) to travel forward.

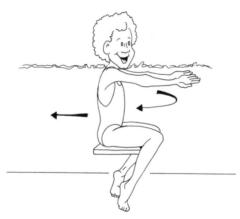

- Use butterflies to travel backward.

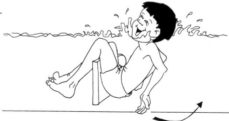

- Kneel on the kickboard and try to travel as described previously.

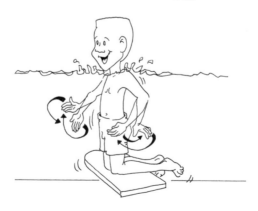

- Lie on the board and surf forward using the crawlstroke or breaststroke.

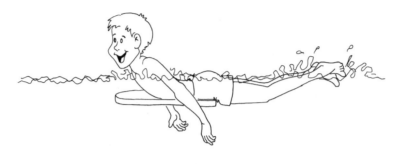

Safety
Be sure that all participants control the board if they slip off during the skill. The board may rocket out of the water and hit an unsuspecting participant. Allow only strong swimmers to travel into deep water on the kickboard.

NOODLE LOCOMOTION

Objectives
Balance and coordination; floating, gliding, and kicking; cardiorespiratory endurance; interval training

Equipment
One noodle per participant

Description
Wrap the noodle around your body at water level so that you can hold on to the ends in your hands. Perform independent locomotor skills as listed in chapter 2 on page 6 and try the following variations:

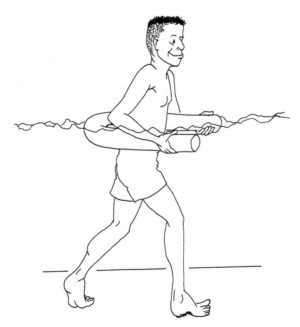

- Jog forward with the noodle wrapped around your trunk. The arms come only to the surface of the water.

- Do supported kicking on your back. Wrap the noodle around your back and lean back on it to support the legs. Use a flutter kick or bicycle kick.

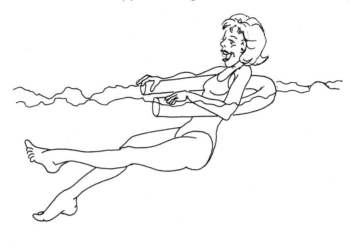

TARZAN SWIM

Objectives
Confidence; independent horizontal motion; crawlstroke; muscular endurance

Equipment
One noodle per participant

Description
Place the noodle across your chest and under your arms. Facing forward, use the noodle for support and swim the crawlstroke, head up.

Safety
Do not let nonswimmers swim into the deep water.

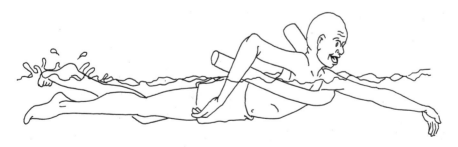

TANDEM NOODLE SKI

Objectives
Cardiorespiratory endurance; interval training; muscular endurance in the triceps

Equipment
One noodle per participant

Description
Partners face the same direction, each holding one end of the noodle, and perform the cross-country ski motion as described in chapter 4. Pull the noodles under the water using the triceps curl.

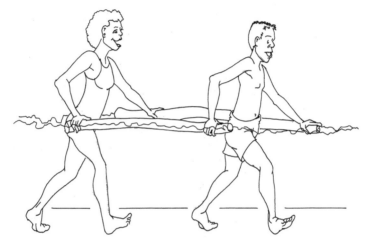

Variations
- Try traveling forward or backward. When moving backward, make sure the space is clear before you move.
- *Tug-of-war:* Face opposite directions and try to pull each other forward.

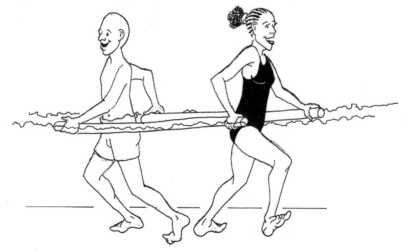

NOODLE BICYCLE

Objectives
Cardiorespiratory endurance; interval training; muscular endurance in the hamstrings and glutei

Equipment
One noodle per participant

Description
Wrap the noodle behind your back and under your arms. Lie on your side and pretend to ride a bicycle. You should travel in a circle. Repeat the motion on the other side.

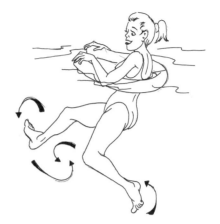

TANDEM BICYCLE

Objectives
Cardiorespiratory endurance; interval training; muscular endurance in the hamstrings

Equipment
One noodle per participant

Description
Partners wrap the noodle behind their backs interlacing them with each other and assume the starting position described in Noodle Bicycle. They bicycle the same direction, pretending to chase each other. On a signal, they reverse direction.

Variation
Combine this exercise with a supported flutter kick. Partners sit back to back, then try to outkick each other. The flutter kick works the quadriceps and the bicycle works the hamstrings to produce good muscle balance.

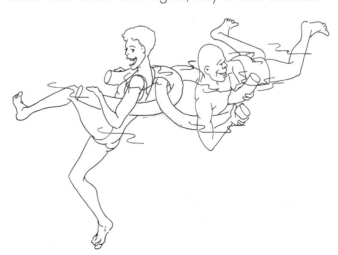

TANDEM NOODLE JACKS

Objective
Add additional resistance to the workout to improve muscular endurance

Equipment
One noodle per participant

Description
Stand facing your partner, each of you holding one end of the noodle. Perform a jumping jack, pulling the noodle underwater in front of you.

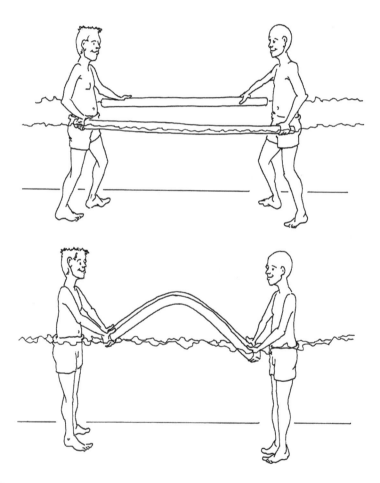

Variations
- Pull the arms behind the body.
- Face the same direction. Partner A pulls the noodle behind while partner B pulls the noodle in front of the body. Try to travel forward, sideways, or backward.

PUSH ME, PULL YOU

Objectives
Interval training; muscular endurance in the upper body

Equipment
One noodle per two participants (two noodles per pair might be needed if participants do not float very well using only one)

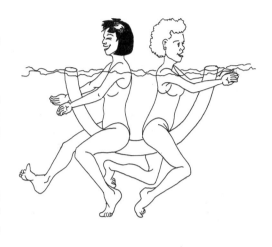

Description
Partners straddle the noodle, sitting back to back, then try to pull away from each other using the breaststroke pull.

Variations
- Race with both partners facing the same direction.
- Sit back to back and have one person pull breaststroke while the other does butterflies.

Relays

The standard relay formation is called a *shuttle* and consists of two boundaries (generally, the side or end walls of the pool). Teams of two, four, or six players are positioned with half of the team at each boundary. The relay proceeds with each participant on the team completing his distance (or *leg*) before the next person begins her distance. (See figure below.) The winner of the relay is the first team whose members have all completed their legs of the race. Organize the relay event using the width of the pool in water 5 feet (1.5 meters) deep or less, or, with swimming variations, using the length of the pool.

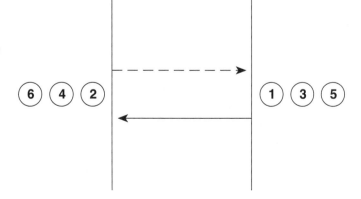

Most of the relays described in this section have swimming variations and will not be repeated in chapter 6 with the swimming stunts, skills, and games. Some of the games contain variations that pair a swimmer with a participant who cannot or chooses not to swim. These "mixed-pairs" activities and skills are described in the swimming chapter but are appropriate for nonswimming events if an adaptation will allow participants to keep their heads out of the water.

MEDLEY DASH RELAY

Objectives
Determined by the skills chosen for locomotion; interval training

Number of Participants
Two or more equal teams of four to six players

Description
Use a shuttle relay formation. Each member of the team is assigned a different method of locomotion (for example, jog, jog backward, step sideways, skip, hop, leap). On the signal, the first member of the team completes his leg of the race and tags the second person. The relay continues until all members of the team have completed their leg of the race.

Variations
- Use stunts and skills described earlier in the chapter.
- Add equipment to the relay.

PARTNER RELAY

Objectives
Determined by skills chosen for locomotion; interval training

Number of Participants
Two or more teams of four, six, or eight players

Description
All members of the team are positioned on the same end or side of the pool. Each team member must have a partner. Each pair completes two legs of the race. One leg is completed with one partner in the lead. At the boundary, the other person takes the lead to finish the second leg. With four members on a team, there are four legs of the race; with six members there are six legs of the race; and so on. The winning team is the one that completes all legs of the race in the fastest time.

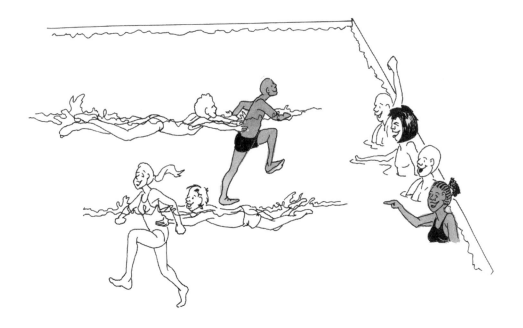

SOCK AND SHIRT RELAY

Objectives
Determined by skills chosen for locomotion; interval training

Number of Participants
Two or more equal teams of four to six players

Equipment
One shirt and one sock per team

Description
Divide the teams as for a shuttle relay. On the signal, the first member of the team puts on the sock and shirt and finishes her leg of the race. She must remove the clothing and give it to the second person, who puts it on before completing his leg. The relay continues until all members of the team have successfully completed the distance wearing the sock and shirt. You may include a rule that allows team members to help each other don the clothes.

Variations
- Use oversized sweatshirts for stronger participants.
- Use additional clothing (for example, two socks, a shoe, a hat, and shorts). Each person must don the previous swimmer's pieces of clothing and add a piece before completing her leg of the relay. The last person to swim is dressed with all of the clothing used in the game.

- Make it a swimming relay.
- Have individuals race against each other rather than race in teams.
- Organize the race in heats determined by the number of lanes available. Each individual has a sock and shirt. On the signal, participants put on the sock and complete the first leg of the race. They climb out of the pool and put on the shirt and then complete the last leg of the race. The winners of each heat race each other in the last heat of the race.

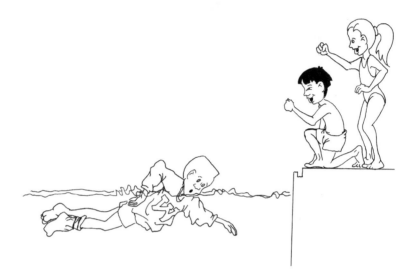

BALLOON RELAY

Objective
Determined by the method chosen for locomotion; interval training

Number of Participants
Two or more equal teams of four to six players

Equipment
One balloon per member of a team, plus extra balloons (start with the balloons blown up and tied)

Description
Organize the teams as for a shuttle relay. On the signal, the first person tucks his balloon under his arm and runs the first leg of the relay. He must pop the balloon before the second person in the relay begins her leg of the race. The relay continues until all members of the team have completed their leg of the race and the balloons are popped.

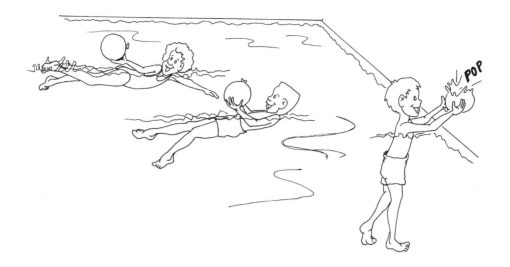

Variations

- Participants must hop out of the water and sit on the balloon to pop it.
- Participants start with a deflated balloon and must blow it up and tie it before entering the pool. (Hint: the bigger they inflate the balloon, the easier it is to pop.)
- More skilled participants may be able to blow the balloon up underwater, tie it off, and then begin the race.
- Select different methods of locomotion to complete each leg of the race to make it a medley relay and/or adapt for participants with different strengths.
- Make it a swimming relay.

Safety

Participants may begin in the water or on deck. If starting from the deck, do not allow headfirst (dive) entries. Always gather remaining balloon pieces when the event is over to keep them from going through the pool filtration system.

RICKSHAW RELAY

Objective
Interval training

Number of Participants
Limited only by the size of the playing area

Equipment
One noodle per two participants

Description
Use a shuttle relay format. Each person needs a partner. Partner A wraps the noodle around the torso at water level. Partner B stands behind A and grabs the ends of the noodle (one end in each hand). Partner B leans backward to get her feet off the bottom of the pool and pretends to ride a rickshaw while A pulls her across the playing area. At the boundary, partners switch places and complete the second leg of the race.

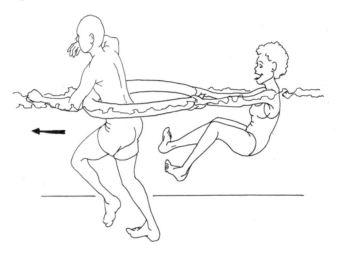

Variations
- *Chariot race:* Partners stand back to back. Wrap the noodle around the trailing partner (partner B) so that partner A can grab the ends of the noodle. Partner A jogs to the boundary pulling partner B. Depending on the strength and the skill of the class, B could do the flutter kick to assist A during the race.

- *Team relay:* With limited equipment, organize the class in teams of four, six, or eight and run the shuttle format. Participants hand the noodle off to the next participants at the boundary. The relay continues until all participants have played partner A and partner B.

Tag Games

Tag games are always exciting but may or may not satisfy the criteria for being interval training. Sometimes the playing area is too small and the game ends too quickly for some participants to work hard, and sometimes the playing area is too large, which allows some players to hide out on the periphery and stand still instead of actively participate. You will need to determine whether these games or variations can be played successfully to meet the fitness goal. On the other hand, all of these games are fun, and fun is certainly an appropriate objective in a fitness class.

FLAG TAG

Objectives
Interval training; muscular endurance, depending on the form of locomotion selected for the game

Number of Participants
Limited only by the size of the playing area

Equipment
One flag football belt (preferably plastic) with two flags per participant

Description
One player is "It." It tries to pull the flags from other participants. Anyone who has both flags pulled becomes another It. The last person to have both flags pulled is It for the next game.

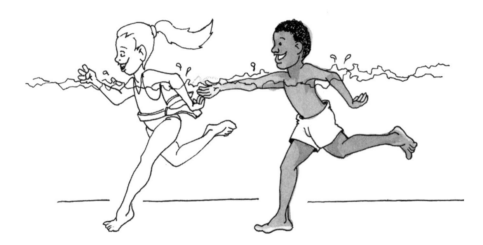

Variations
- Designate the method of locomotion (jog, skip, or walk backward, for example).
- *Team Flag Tag:* Form two equal teams. One team wears the flags, and the other team is It. Teams line up on opposite sides of the pool. On the signal, the flag team tries to reach the other boundary before all flags are pulled. The flag team receives a point for each person who makes it across the pool with at least one flag intact. Players who cross the pool with both flags intact get two points. The flag team becomes It for the second game. The team with the most points at the end of an even number of games is declared the winner.
- If there are enough good swimmers in the group, use the whole pool and divide it into deep and shallow games.

Safety
Players must not climb ladders or get out of the pool to escape It.

FUSION TAG

Objective
Interval training

Number of Participants
Limited only by the size of the playing area

Description
One person is designated as It. All other participants line up against one boundary, and It stands between them and the other boundary. On the signal, all participants run to the other boundary. It tags someone, and the two become fused into a pair (by linking elbows). Each member of the pair must now try to tag someone with his free hand. When each member of the pair has tagged another participant, the four fused together split into two pairs. Now there are two Its. Participants who reach the boundary without getting tagged continue to run from one boundary to the other until all players have been paired off.

Variations
- Play without boundaries so there are no "safe" areas.
- For continuous play, the last person to be tagged becomes It for the next game.

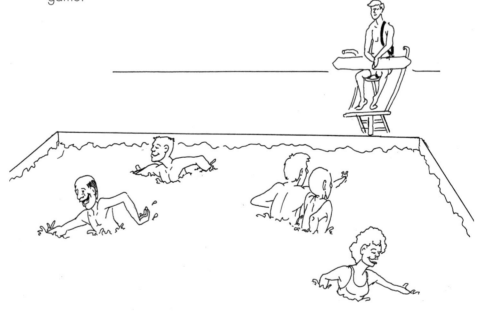

PINBALL TAG

Objective
Interval training

Number of Participants
Limited only by the size of the playing area

Description
One person for every 10 players is designated as It (for example, with 30 players, 3 people are It). All other participants line up on one boundary. It stands between them and the other boundary. (Use the sides of the pool for boundaries.) The object of the game is for participants to cross back and forth to reach the boundaries five times without being touched by It. If they are touched by It as they try to cross to the next boundary, they must return to the boundary from which they came and start the lap over.

The first person to finish five laps (one lap is one time across) is the winner and becomes It for the next game. If playing with multiple Its, when the first participant completes five laps, have him select other Its to begin the new game.

Variations
- Vary the method of locomotion with each game.
- Use swimming strokes.

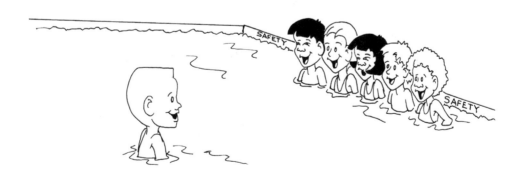

Individual and Team Events

The games in this section do not fall neatly into the categories already described, although some of them can be done relay style. Many of them do not require enough exertion to be considered for intervals, but they are certainly appropriate for warm-up, cool-down, and active recovery phases of the workout.

FOLLOW THE LEADER

Objective
Appropriate for all phases of the workout depending on the fitness objective

Number of Participants
Limited only by the size of the playing area

Description
Select a pattern of organization that is appropriate for the play area and the number of participants. (See examples under Variations.) Designate a leader. The leader demonstrates the skill and then leads the participants through the pattern of organization or for a designated number of repetitions. Each participant takes a turn

at being leader. To create intervals, use a signal to speed up play for a predetermined interval. Then let the new leader determine the activity for the active recovery phase.

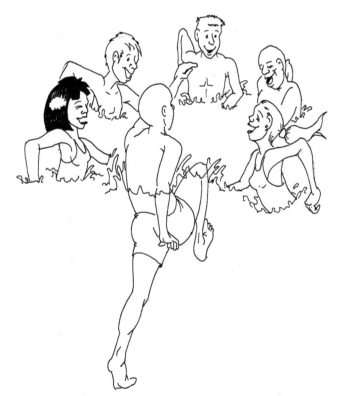

Variations
- *Circle:* Each leader leads a predetermined number of repetitions or is given a time limit (30 to 60 seconds max) to complete a skill set. Rotate around the circle with a new leader after each interval.

- *Line:* Line up participants against one boundary. The leader moves across the playing area to the second boundary and the participants follow performing the skill. Select a new leader at each boundary.

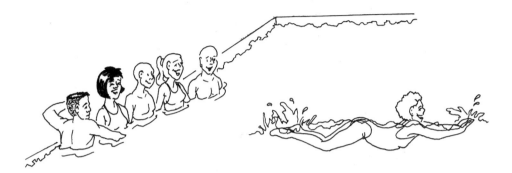

- Play partner stunts follow the leader. Each person pairs up with another player and the two choose a partner activity to lead. Pairs move through the designated format following the lead pair's lead. Use the partner activities previously described in this chapter.

Safety
For comfort and security, do not allow leaders to choose swimming options if some participants are unwilling to attempt them.

OBJECT RETRIEVAL RACE

Objectives
Confidence in the water; independent locomotion; interval training

Number of Participants
Two or more equally numbered teams

Equipment
One plastic container for each team (large drink cup or plastic cereal bowl, for example); many small floating objects (different sizes of corks, Ping-Pong balls, plastic golf balls, or old noodles cut into sections small enough to grab easily)

Description
Place the plastic containers around the playing area to mark boundaries. Teams remain at their boundaries until play begins. Throw all the floating objects into the pool. On the signal, team members retrieve one object at a time and return it to their team's container. The winning team is the one with the most floating objects in their container.

Participants may swim or run back to the container. If they are allowed to use swimming strokes, which are faster and more efficient, be sure that there are equal numbers of swimmers on each team to keep one team from gaining an advantage. You can also restrict the method of locomotion to swimming only or running only, or use alternative forms of locomotion depending on the skill level of the group and the fitness focus.

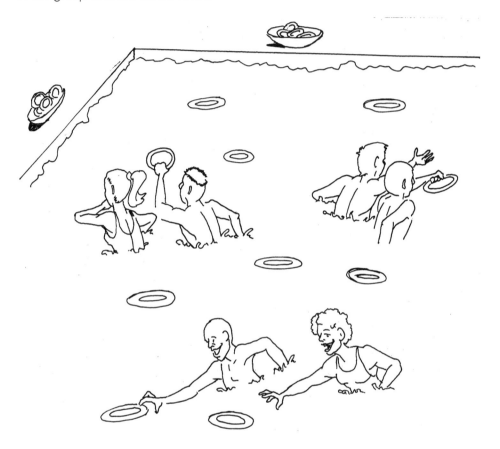

Variations

- Number the members of each team consecutively by ones (1, 2, and so on) or by twos if the teams have more than four people. Throw an object into the pool between the teams (equidistant from each). Call out a number. All members with that number jump into the water, race to the object, and try to bring it back to their team. If there are two teams, use one object. If there are three teams, use two objects, and so on. Each team member may retrieve only one object for the team. To speed up the pace of the game, throw in more objects and call out more than one number at a time. The winner is the team that collects the most objects.

- Divide the group into two teams and have the teams line up on opposite sides of the pool. Throw as many objects into the water as there are participants in the game. Run the game relay style. On the signal, one player from each team retrieves an object and takes it back to the team. Each player follows in succession, retrieving an object, until all players have an object. The winner is the team who can complete the task in the shortest amount of time.

- Use coins so that participants must go underwater to retrieve the object. Pennies count for one point. Each silver coin is worth its value in points for the team. Silver money is harder to see. Swimmers will have to stay underwater longer and search closer to the bottom to see the silver coins.

- Take old noodles that have been cut in small sections and use a permanent marker to write letters on each piece. Each team is given a word to spell. Participants retrieve letters to spell their word. Points are awarded for speed and correct spelling.

PIGEON RACE

Objectives
Independent locomotion; interval training

Number of Participants
Limited only by the size of the playing area

Description
Participants line up on one side of the pool. On the signal, they race to the other side of the pool and hop out to sit on the edge using a pool push-up. Points are awarded to the person who is the first to get seated on the side of the pool. Participants continue racing back and forth between boundaries until they have covered a certain distance or crossed a predetermined number of times, or a certain amount of time has elapsed, or one participant earns a certain number of total points. (If the coping or gutter system will not accommodate quick exit, select a pose or position for the "pigeons" to perform on completion of the race.)

Variations
- Select different methods of locomotion (for example, run, bob, skip, hop, hold on to one leg and hop, swim with one arm, step sideways).

- Select more than one winner. Winners sit out one race, then rejoin the game.

- Use the Whistle Stop Stunt Race as a format (see page 101).

- *Partner Pigeon:* Use the partner skills described earlier in the chapter. For example, use the chariot race previously described on page 90 to travel from boundary to boundary.

- *Team Pigeon:* Organize in teams of equal numbers. Use a shuttle relay format. The team with all the pigeons on the deck in the least amount of time is the winner.
- Play in deep water. Swimmers will need more room to keep from running into each other. Do not use underwater swimming as an option for completing the distance of the relay.

Safety
Arrange the class so that taller people are in deeper water. Everyone should be in or near chest-deep water. Make sure all students have enough room to jump in at the start and enough room to use the arms during the race. Check the pool deck for any sharp areas at the boundary line if participants will hop out to finish the race.

MUSICAL NOODLES OR KICKBOARDS

Objectives
Dynamic balance; cardiorespiratory endurance

Number of Participants
Limited by the size of the playing area and the number of noodles or kickboards available

Equipment
One less noodle or kickboard than the number of participants in the game; some form of music that can be stopped and started quickly

Description
Form a circle. Place all the equipment in the center of the circle. As the music plays, the participants walk or run around the circle in the same direction. When the music stops, all participants grab a piece of equipment. The person who ends up without the noodle or board has to walk around the outside of the circle of other players in the opposite direction during the next musical series. Remove a noodle or board after each series until there is only one for the last two players. Eventually, there will be more players in the outside circle than in the inside circle playing the game. Keep the players in the outside circle moving, cheering, and involved.

Variations
- Have good swimmers play in deep water.
- *Musical Duck and Dive:* Use nonbuoyant objects instead of boards so that players must duck under the water to retrieve an object off the bottom of the pool when the music stops. For safety, spread the objects out on the bottom to avoid collisions. Use this variation with good swimmers in deep water.

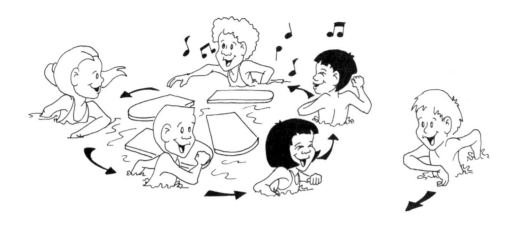

Safety
Remember that moving water can knock unsuspecting participants off their feet. Do not allow the circle to get so large that participants are in danger of drifting into deeper water.

TUG-OF-WAR

Objective
Interval training

Number of Participants
Two teams of 6 to 10 players

Equipment
3/4-inch nylon rope the length of the playing area; a bright-colored heavy plastic bottle; two markers for the pool bottom (rubber bases or traffic cones [pylons] work well)

Description
Tie the bottle at the midpoint of the rope. Set the markers on the pool bottom, 6 to 10 feet (2 to 3 meters) apart and equidistant from the two boundaries. Use standard rules for tug-of-war. The winner is the team to pull the bottle past its marker.

Variation
Swimmers can play tug-of-war in deep water. An official will need to stand in line with the pool markers to determine when one team has met the objective.

Safety
Do not allow participants to wrap the rope around their bodies. Participants may want to wear cotton gloves to avoid rope burns.

FILL THE HOLE

Objective
Warm-up or cool-down

Number of Participants
Minimum of 6 (12 to 20 per group preferred)

Description
Form a circle. Count off by fours (for larger groups, count off by fives or sixes). Depending on the age of the participants in the group, you can use numbers, letters, or names to identify each group (1s are seals, 2s are turtles, and so on). One person is designated as It and goes into the center of the circle. It calls out the name of one of the groups. On the signal, each member of that group changes places with another person from the same group. It tries to fill a hole left by one of the members of the group. The person who cannot find a hole in the circle becomes the new It.

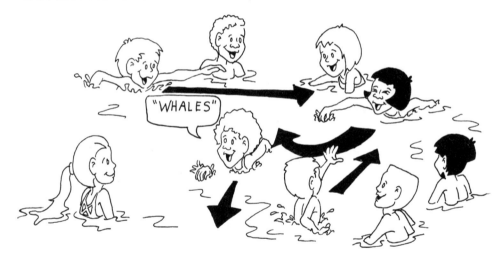

Variations
- Change the method of traveling to the new place in the circle (for example, swim a stroke, walk backward, or skip).
- To challenge swimmers and improve fitness, play in deep water.

BEACH BALL VOLLEYBALL

Objectives
Socialization; eye–hand coordination; vertical jump; cardiorespiratory endurance

Number of Participants
Two evenly numbered teams, limited only by the size of the playing area

Equipment
Beach ball and a rope or net to divide the playing area in half; in a pool with lane lines, move all of the lines together to divide the pool by its length.

Description
Use standard volleyball rules, but prohibit spiking and dunking. With large classes and limited pool space, allow part of the team to sit on the boundary (edge of the pool) and keep the ball in play. Rotate the group in the water and out of the water every one to three minutes.

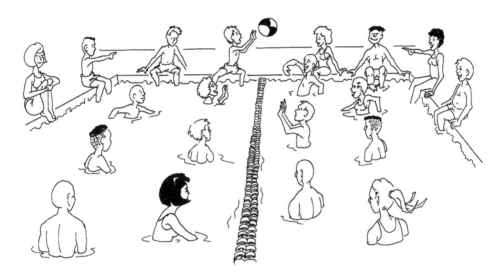

Variations
- Specify more than three hits on a side.
- Use only two-handed overhead passes.
- If you have a heavy volleyball net, place a sheet over the netted area so that teams cannot see the ball coming.
- Challenge swimmers to play in the deep end and tread water.

WHISTLE STOP STUNT RACE

Objectives
Determined by stunts selected for the game; interval training

Number of Participants
Limited only by the size of the playing area

Description
Establish two different boundaries. All participants line up at one boundary. Participants race toward the opposite boundary using a predetermined method of independent locomotion or partner stunt (for example, hop, run, partner tow,

skip, or jog backward). When participants are approximately halfway to the boundary, blow a whistle. On the whistle, participants must stop, complete a predetermined number of repetitions of the skill chosen for this activity, and then race to the boundary. The winner sits out one race and then rejoins for the next series.

Variations

- Use partner stunts (for example, power knee lifts, rebounds, swing your partner, jump a half-turn).
- Use a team of three or four. One team goes at a time. Each team forms a float pattern or letter. (See chapter 6, page 139, for an explanation of float patterns.) Teams are timed for the whistle stop stunt, and the winning team is the team with the fastest time.
- Challenge swimmers with stunts and skills described in chapter 6 (front flip, back flip, handstand, kip, log roll, bob, tub turn, and the like).

SURVIVOR CHALLENGE

Objectives
Determined by the objectives of the skills chosen for the event; interval training

Prerequisites
Independent locomotion; aqua basics

Number of Participants
Two or more teams of four to six players (size of the teams determines the length of the work phase of the interval set)

Equipment
Challenge cards (One set for each team, one card per each player on the team; write on each card the name of the aqua basic skill and the number of repetitions needed to complete the set. If you laminate the cards, they can be reused.)

Description
Establish two boundaries. They do not have to be ends of the pool. All teams start at one boundary. The challenge cards are placed at the second boundary. On the signal to start, one member from each team runs to the second boundary and retrieves a challenge card and brings it back to the team. All team members must complete the challenge on the card at the same time. Another member of the team takes the challenge card back to the boundary and retrieves a different card. The game proceeds until all challenges have been completed.

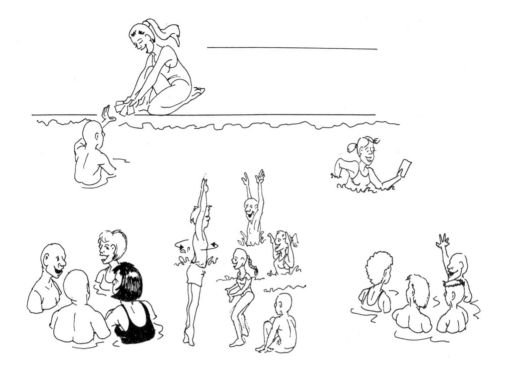

Variations

- Have each team submit one activity for the challenge.
- Add another challenge: All teams must return to the second boundary after the last challenge card and then complete all challenges without a break to win the game. If you use this variation, limit team size to two to four people so the work interval is manageable.

This activity is adapted from a presentation made at 2004 AAHPERD Convention. "Athletic Aqua." Presenters were Karen Dyer, M.S., ACE, AEA and Susan McDonald ACE, AEA, Vanderbilt University.

WAVE GAUNTLET

Objectives
Muscular endurance of the chest and upper-back muscles; interval training

Number of Participants
Limited only by the size of the playing area, but more participants create more wave action

Equipment
One kickboard per participant

Description

Form two equal lines of participants facing each other. Using the chest pass with the kickboard, they push the water toward each other, creating a wave gauntlet. Two at a time, participants challenge the gauntlet by moving down the line between the waves, working with the kickboard to stay balanced. When the first two participants get about halfway through the gauntlet, the next pair begins. As they finish the gauntlet, each pair joins the wave-making machine and the activity continues until all participants have challenged the gauntlet. If the group is large, you may have to give the upper-body muscles a break and do the wave gauntlet as interval sets.

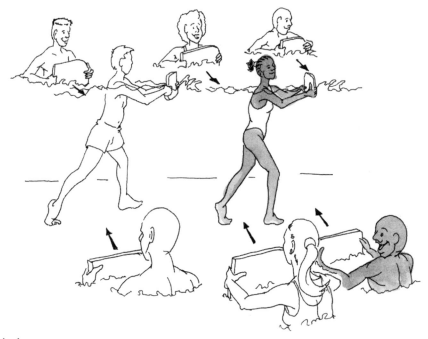

Variations

- Organize the wave machine in a circle to challenge balance and core stability.
- Divide the group into two teams. One team forms the wave gauntlet and the other team swims the gauntlet, one swimmer at a time. Then teams trade positions.

Safety

Have participants stand far enough from each other that they do not hit those challenging the gauntlet with their kickboards.

HYDRO-TRIATHLON

Objectives
Cardiorespiratory endurance or interval training, depending on the distance for each of the three parts of the triathlon; muscular endurance, depending on the activities selected for the event.

Number of Participants
Limited only by the size of the playing area

Equipment
Optional for variations (kickboards or noodles)

Description
Establish the boundaries or mark a course for the event. Select three different forms of locomotion. These should work different muscle groups so that there is some muscular rest between each leg of the event. On the signal, participants move from boundary to boundary around the course, changing the method of locomotion at each boundary. The person with the fastest time wins.

Variations
- *Partners:* Do the activity using some form of partner locomotion.
- *Team tri:* Teams of three have two boundaries. One participant is at one boundary and two participants are at the other boundary. Run as a shuttle format, with one of the two participants beginning the race. Each participant completes one leg of the race, each doing a different form of locomotion. If there are enough swimmers for each team to have one, swim a leg, run a leg, and then select one other activity to finish the triathlon.
- If you want to use this event for cardiorespiratory endurance, run it as a continuous shuttle—A races to B, B races to C, C races to A, and then they begin again. Each time they start over, they have to do a different event. Continue the event for the predetermined cardiorespiratory endurance set, or set up interval training using this same format.
- *Kickboards:* Use one board per team of three participants. Run the event as a shuttle relay. Each person completes a leg using a kickboard (for example, flutter kick, sit on the board, and swim breaststroke).
- *Noodles:* Same as the kickboard variation, racing with the noodle (for example, tuck it under your arms and paddle crawlstroke, wrap it around your torso and run, sit on it between your legs and breaststroke).

Sample Games Workout

To help you put this all together, here's a sample workout you might create using some of the activities we've seen so far.

Workout segment	Activities	Time for activity/ Elapsed time in minutes
Warm-up	Big Circle–Little Circle (chapter 4)	5/5
Precardio	Follow the Leader (circle formation)	5/10
Cardiorespiratory endurance	Rope jumps combined with front kicks, side kicks, mountain climbers, cross-country ski, butt kickers, jumping jacks	7/17
Interval set	Medley Dash (chapter 5)	3/20
Cardiorespiratory endurance	Repeat the first cardiorespiratory endurance set	7/27
Interval set	Pinball Tag (chapter 5)	3/30
Cardiorespiratory endurance	Repeat the first cardiorespiratory endurance set	7/37
Interval set	Repeat Medley Dash with new teams	3/40
Cool-down	Big Circle–Little Circle format with easy stretch and range-of-motion activities	10/50

chapter 6

Swimming Activities and Games

If you have been successful with the shallow-water games and activities, you have probably noticed that participants now display more courage in attempting skills that simulate swimming skills (any skill that involves a horizontal position, supported or unsupported). Now it is time to encourage them to give swimming skills a try. With the help of the Swim Activity Finder, you can choose the water adjustment activities, stunts and skills, swimming games, and fitness swimming formats that work best for your class.

Before we move on, however, let's learn an assessment process that will help you evaluate your participants' readiness. It's important not to rush people into doing an activity that makes them anxious. So slow down, take your time, and enjoy the trip.

Assessing Readiness

In order to select appropriate activities, you should have a pretty good idea of the skill level of your group. It is not unusual to have good swimmers and nonswimmers participating in the same group or activity. You should provide some form of skill assessment before you begin your activity or program. One of the easiest and least-threatening ways to accomplish this is to use a stunt circle activity.

The *stunt circle* is a quick, safe, nonthreatening approach to assessing the water adjustment and swimming skills of your group. No swimming skills are necessary, and participants do not have to get their faces wet to participate unless they want to.

Organize the group in one large circle in standing-depth water (chest deep, if possible). Have participants count off by twos (1, 2, 1, 2, and so on). If the number in the circle is even, stand outside the circle and give directions; if the number is uneven, you will need to join the circle during the assessment.

To set up the circle for assessment, have the 1s support the 2s. The 1s keep their feet on the bottom of the pool using a wide base of support (feet shoulder-width apart and knees bent slightly). They support by reaching under the arms and across the backs of the 2s on either side of them. The assessment begins with the 2s doing supported front and back floats in the circle. Give directions using a movement exploration format: "Who can do [name a movement]?"

Have the group attempt the following skills:

- Front float with face out of the water (feet should be on the surface outside the circle)
- Front float, face out, and flutter kick
- Nose bubbles with eyes above the surface (see more on nose bubbles on page 111)
- Front float, face in, to the count of 3, 4, or 5
- Front float, face in, and kick
- Back float with feet on the surface (participants will have feet on the inside of the circle)
- Back float and kick
- Back float with ears wet
- Back float, ears wet, and kick

Make a mental note of students who seem apprehensive: those who will not submerge on the front float; those who will not get their ears wet on the back float; and those who continue to move, wiggle, or thrash about even when the skill should be performed motionless. Then have the 2s support and the 1s try the skills.

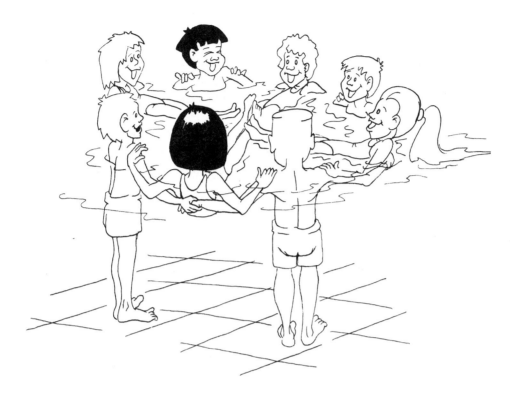

After completing this, try the circle again with a new challenge. Instead of supporting with the arms across the back, have the participants hold hands. Challenge the participants to let go of hands during the skills whenever possible. Identify those who cannot do skills unsupported. Later you can fill in the skills assessment checklist found in appendix D to help identify students' needs. Use the activity finder to select games that are appropriate to the skills of the group as a whole.

Select activities that are age and skill appropriate. The younger the participant, the less complex the games should be. Be sure that all participants possess the prerequisite skills necessary to successfully engage in the game, stunt, or skill. If not all participants can be successful as the activity is written, use your imagination to create a variation of the game.

Using the Swim Activity Finder

The Swim Activity Finder, like the Fitness Activity Finder, is at the beginning of this book. The Swim Activity Finder is arranged so that, at a glance, you can find the appropriate stunt, skill, activity, or game based on the skill levels within your group. The activities (Activity type) are classified as water adjustment, stunts and skills, swimming games, or fitness swimming.

Prerequisite skills are provided to help you measure the difficulty of the activity. These prerequisites include independent locomotion (see chapter 2, page 6), submersion, unsupported floating and gliding, sculling, and swimming skills. We also have included additional skills that are necessary for safe and comfortable swimming experiences.

Beginning swimmers are often apprehensive about putting their faces in the water or trusting that they can stay on the surface of the water and not sink. These skills are especially stressful for people who have, at some time in their lives, had a bad experience with water (such as almost drowning, feeling that they would drown, or seeing someone else drown). For this reason, you need to guide them slowly through the new experiences that will help them relax and enjoy the water. These skills are progressive, meaning that they build off each other and are necessary to continue to progress through the learning stages. Many of them are listed as prerequisites for participation in the games and activities in this chapter.

Submerging

Putting the face in the water can be a frightening experience. There are so many new sensations when you completely submerge. The water may initially sting your eyes. Water that goes up the nose causes an unpleasant burning sensation, and, for some people, water in the ears may cause dizziness. All of these feelings are normal and common, and with time and a few hints from you, your participants will learn to be comfortable and relaxed with submersion. The following are keys to mastering the submersion skill.

Breath Control

Learning good breath control is the key to comfortable and relaxed swimming. Breath control involves the ability to hold your breath as well as to properly exchange air through your mouth and nose in a rhythmic manner. Rhythmic air exchange refers to inhaling through the mouth and exhaling underwater through the mouth and nose. Exhaling through the nose should be emphasized in the early stages of learning to decrease the chances of inhaling water up the nose (not a very pleasant feeling).

Without ever putting the face in the water, participants can learn to exhale through the nose by pretending to blow the nose into a hanky. Place the hands gently over the nose to cover it as if using a hanky. In chest-deep water, lean forward until the palms begin to touch the water and exhale into your "hanky." The air that comes out of your nose will make bubbles in the water.

An alternative method of exhaling through the nose is simply to hum, which forces air out of the nose and prevents water from entering. Begin with the chin on the surface of the water. Take a breath, close the lips, and begin humming. Slowly lower the face until the nostrils are just under the surface of the water. The eyes are still out of the water. Humming with the nose submerged makes *nose bubbles*. (To practice air exchange with a partner, see the Teeter-Totter activity later in this chapter.) Participants should inhale through the mouth only. Remind them that when they come up out of the water, water drips from the hair and face and is easily inhaled into the nose if one is not careful (again, not a pleasant experience).

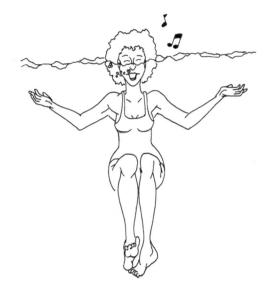

Breath Holding

Swimming strokes and skills don't require long periods of breath holding, but participants should be comfortable holding their breath for 5 to 10 seconds to enjoy underwater activities. You may wonder how they can hold their breath when they are blowing nose bubbles. If they blow bubbles as the nose first enters the water, the air is trapped in the nostrils. At this point they can stop blowing and the air in the nostrils blocks the water from getting in. If they exhale through the nose just before coming up, they will be ready to inhale through the mouth.

The breath-holding skill comes with an added precaution: Participants should avoid extended breath holding and a process known as *hyperventilation.* Hyperventilation is taking a series of long breaths in an effort to extend breath-holding time. This process blows off the carbon dioxide in your system that triggers your breathing response. Without carbon dioxide in your brain, you will not feel the urge to breathe. The problem arises when you hold your breath underwater after hyperventilating. Without the urge to breathe, you don't have oxygen in your system and you black out. If you black out underwater, you will inhale water and possibly drown.

To avoid the consequences of hyperventilation, discuss the dangers with your group and be watchful during underwater activities. Do not allow participants to take more than one or two long, deep breaths before submerging. Do not allow breath-holding contests or swimming underwater for distance.

Underwater Sight

Seeing underwater is a unique and exciting experience. At first the eyes might sting a bit, but participants will quickly adjust and have little trouble seeing objects or other participants. Seeing underwater reduces the chance of collisions with other swimmers or with the side of the pool. It also provides swimmers with important kinesthetic feedback about where their bodies are during an activity.

Though being able to open the eyes underwater without protection (goggles or mask) is an important safety skill, people who are apprehensive about submersion may benefit from using a mask or goggles. Participants who have not mastered nose bubbles should use a mask to improve confidence. Switch them to goggles after they master nose bubbles. Goggles are also appropriate for individuals who wear contacts.

If participants will spend the majority of the activity time with eyes open underwater, they should be encouraged to wear goggles to reduce eye irritation. For safety, be sure that participants do not submerge more than 3 to 4 feet (about 1 meter) using the goggles because water pressure on the goggles can damage the soft tissue around the eyes. For more information on using goggles, refer to appendix A.

Recovery to a Stand

Before practicing unsupported floating or gliding, participants should be shown how to return to a standing position. You can use a noodle to facilitate independent practice, and participants do not need to submerge.

Place both hands in the center of the noodle and extend it in front of you as you push off into a front glide. To recover to a stand, pull down on the noodle and pull the knees toward the chest at the same time. When the knees are near the noodle, extend the legs to touch the feet on the bottom. Instructors can assist by supporting the noodle as necessary. When the participant can float or glide independently, allow him to recover on his own. (See lead-up skills, pages 28 to 29).

Unsupported Floating or Gliding

The ability to float or glide a short distance without support is an important step toward independent swimming. Once participants can relax on their front or back and use the water for support, they will begin to experience success in swimming strokes. The prone float or glide requires facedown breath holding. Extend the arms over the head, put the face in the water, and slowly lift the feet off the pool bottom to float (push with the feet to glide forward).

The back float should be started in chest-deep water with the arms extended horizontally to the side. Take a deep breath and put the head back in the water until the ears are wet. Relax and let the feet float off the bottom of the pool. It is not necessary for participants to float in a horizontal position. The key is to maintain an unsupported float for 3 to 5 seconds. Recovering from a back float or glide is as simple as sitting down in a chair. Pull a chair under the buttocks and at the same time

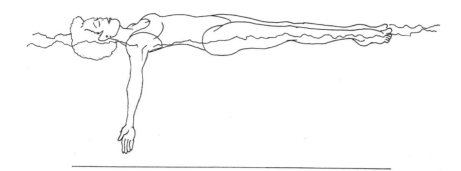

pull the knees toward the chest. Then just stand up. Instructors should assist participants back to a standing position as necessary.

Rolling Over

Mastering the *rollover* skill allows participants to change strokes or to rest after rolling from front to back. To roll from front to back, finish the stroke by bringing an arm down to the side and looking over the same shoulder in the direction of the roll. Take a deep breath as the face comes out of the water and continue swimming on the back.

To roll from back to front, look in the direction of the roll. If rolling left, reach across the chest with the right arm without lifting it out of the water. Reach to a point in front of the head and continue stroking on the front. For a lead-up activity that does not require submersion, see Flip-Flops later in this chapter.

Changing Directions

Changing directions helps you return to the side of the pool or to a position of safety. Participants should be able to swim a short distance away from poolside and return using a wide turn. This is accomplished by looking and stroking harder in the direction of the turn. Another method of changing direction is to stop swimming, tread water, turn and face the new direction, and begin swimming back to poolside.

Treading Water

Treading water is the deep-water support position. Participants who master this skill can enjoy most of the deep-water activities. It is performed in a semi-vertical position, with the head up and out of the water. The arms perform a broad sculling motion. Sculling was first described in chapter 4 as an aqua basic skill to develop muscular endurance in the arms.

Begin with the palms facing the bottom of the pool. With the elbows bent and arms in front of you, move the hands toward each other in front of

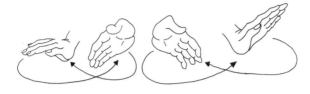

the chest and then away to a position wider than the shoulders. The action is similar to smoothing sand on the beach. The smoothing action creates downward pressure on the water to keep you up. The legs assist by kicking downward. See examples in the figures below. Use a modified bicycle kick, scissors kick (*a-b*), breaststroke kick (*c-d*), or rotary kick (*e*).

Students can practice treading water in shallow water, using only the arms for support. They should work to keep the head out of the water by using broad sculling motions and pulling the legs toward the chest. If swimmers can support themselves using only the arms in this manner, they will be successful using any of the kicks.

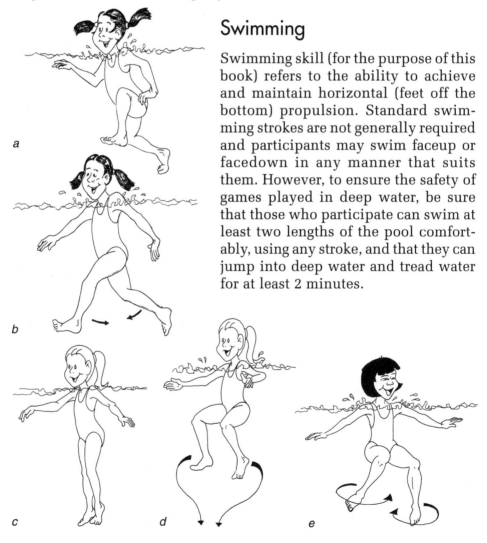

Swimming

Swimming skill (for the purpose of this book) refers to the ability to achieve and maintain horizontal (feet off the bottom) propulsion. Standard swimming strokes are not generally required and participants may swim faceup or facedown in any manner that suits them. However, to ensure the safety of games played in deep water, be sure that those who participate can swim at least two lengths of the pool comfortably, using any stroke, and that they can jump into deep water and tread water for at least 2 minutes.

Whenever you do any of the activities in this chapter, be sure to observe the standard safety precautions for exercise described in chapter 3.

Water Adjustment and Warm-Up Activities

Most of the water adjustment activities are lead-ups to improve readiness for stunts and skills and to practice prerequisite skills for the games and swimming activities later in the chapter. Many of them are perfect for socialization or for the warm-up segment of a fitness workout. The major objective for all these activities is to encourage independent, relaxed participation in the water. Most important, they are self-paced, in order to decrease the anxiety of being compared to other participants.

BLOWING A FLOATING OBJECT

Objectives
Water adjustment; breath control

Prerequisite
Independent locomotion

Number of Participants
Limited only by the size of the playing area

Equipment
Large corks, Ping-Pong balls, or plastic golf balls (one for each participant or pair of participants)

Description
Participants practice blowing the object across the pool as they walk. They may blow the object to a partner who blows it back.

Variation
Do the drill as a shuttle relay.

Safety
Participants can get their mouths very close to the water to blow on the object. Tell participants to tilt their heads back before blowing so they don't inhale water.

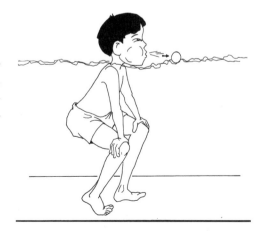

LISTENING UNDERWATER

Objectives
Water adjustment; awareness of senses

Prerequisites
Submersion; breath control

Number of Participants
Limited only by the size of the playing area

Equipment
Objects that make noise (examples: use a metal object to strike a stainless steel ladder in the pool; use a heavy chain to make a rattling noise; use a duck call, whistle, or bell; use both hands to pull the air underwater to make a "whomp" sound that can be heard underwater)

Description
Participants go underwater, listen for the sound, and guess what it is.

Safety
Make sure that the objects you have chosen are safe for the pool.

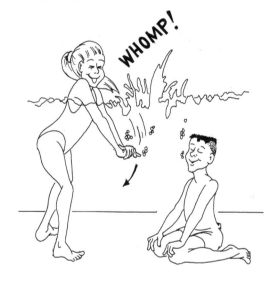

SPLASH THE TEACHER

Objectives
Water adjustment; get wet without going underwater; social interaction

Prerequisite
Independent locomotion

Number of Participants
Limited only by the size of the playing area

Description
Form a circle with the teacher in the center. On the signal, everyone tries to splash the teacher to get her wet. The teacher signals stop by raising her hands in the air. Anyone who does not stop splashing goes to the center of the circle.

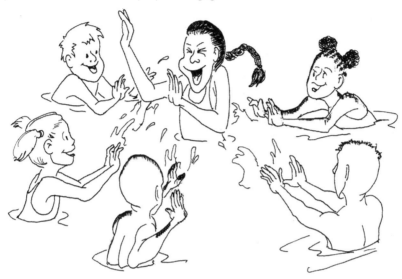

SKY BALL

Objectives
Water adjustment; social interaction; eye-hand coordination; balance

Prerequisites
Independent locomotion

Number of Participants
8 to 10 per circle

Equipment
One beach ball per circle

Description
Form a circle. Throw the beach ball up and have participants try to keep it in the air for as long as possible. Participants may hit with one or both hands, and at various times you can instruct them to hit only with the left hand or only with the right hand. Add rules for older participants, such as no consecutive hits, only one-handed hits, or only overhead hits.

Variation
Let good swimmers play in deep water.

Safety
Do not allow nonswimmers to chase a loose ball into deep water.

HUMAN CORK

Objectives
Water adjustment; motionless front floating; experimenting with buoyancy

Prerequisite
Submersion

Number of Participants
Limited only by the size of the playing area

Description
There are several ways to practice this skill:

- Participants do a supported front float while holding on to the side of the pool. On a signal they let go with the hands for a count of three.
- A buddy pulls his partner in a front glide. On the signal, they try to let go for a count of three.
- Participants take a deep breath and slowly reach down their legs toward the feet. The feet should begin to float up. Challenge the participants to float like a cork a little longer each time they try it.

Safety
- Be sure to pair nonswimmers with someone they can trust.
- Do not exceed 10 seconds of breath holding doing this skill.

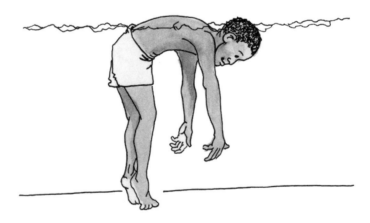

WATER BARREL

Objectives
Water adjustment; stroke mechanics for front crawl, butterfly, or breaststroke

Prerequisites
Independent locomotion; mechanics of the arm strokes

Number of Participants
Limited only by the size of the playing area; minimum of four per circle

Description
Form a circle. Tell participants to pretend that it is a bucket full of water. Use the arm stroke of your choice to pull all the water out of the bucket.

Safety
Participants will travel forward when they pull. Keep the group spread out to avoid collisions.

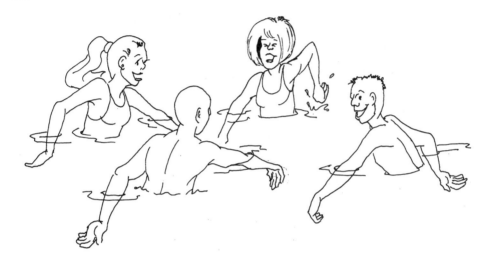

FISH FLOP

Objectives
Water adjustment; unsupported forward propulsion in the prone position (lead-up to butterfly stroke)

Prerequisites
Independent locomotion; submersion optional

Number of Participants
Limited only by the size of the playing area

Description
Stand in chest-deep water. Bend the knees to push off the bottom. Push off with the legs and at the same time reach the arms over the surface as if performing the butterfly stroke. Try to flop, chest first, on the surface of the water so that the feet come out of the water and then splash down on the surface of the water, similar to a dolphin kick. Bend the knees and pull down with the arms to get the feet back on the bottom. Resume a standing position between each fish flop and continue across the pool.

Safety
Be sure that all participants can get back on their feet between fish flops. Everyone should travel in the same direction across the shallow part of the pool.

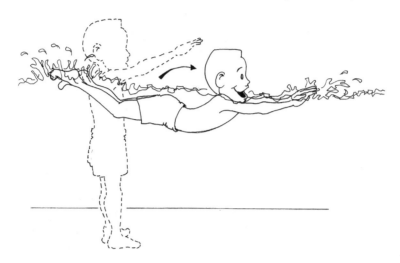

TEETER-TOTTER

Objective
Water adjustment; breath control

Prerequisite
Independent locomotion; submersion

Description
Partners face each other and either hold hands or grasp each other's wrists. One partner goes underwater and exhales through the mouth and nose. As he returns to the surface for another breath, the other partner goes underwater and exhales. It looks like the action of a teeter-totter.

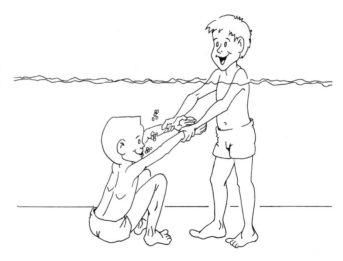

SITTING ON THE BOTTOM

Objectives
Water adjustment; relaxed participation underwater; breath control

Prerequisite
Submersion

Number of Participants
Limited only by the size of the playing area

Description
Begin standing in chest-deep water, bending the knees until the shoulders are wet. Keep arms at the sides, submerge the face, and begin gently exhaling (humming) through the nose to sink down and sit on the bottom of the pool. The legs will be extended in front of the body.

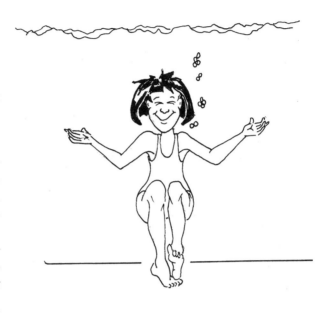

You can get to the bottom faster by using the arms to pull the water up when beginning to descend. As soon as the head submerges, turn the palms up and push hard toward the surface of the water.

LYING ON THE BOTTOM

Objectives
Water adjustment; unsupported submersion; underwater exploration; control of personal buoyancy

Prerequisite
Submersion

Description
Start in a standing position with arms at the sides, palms up. Bend the knees in preparation to jump. Lean forward slightly. Jump up and kick the legs back, lifting the feet off the bottom of the pool. At the same time, push the arms up and

forward to push the body to the bottom, feetfirst. Exhale through the nose and mouth to go down faster. The chest will be the last thing to touch the bottom. To come to the surface, push off the bottom with the hands.

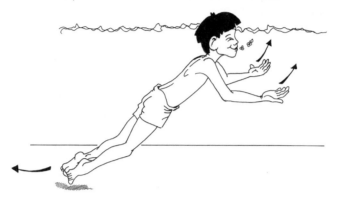

FIRE POLE

Objectives
Water adjustment; supported submersion; underwater exploration; lead-up for deep-water exploration

Prerequisite
Submersion

Number of Participants
Limited only by the size of the playing area and the availability of equipment

Equipment
One reaching pole or rescue pole/shepherd's crook

Description
Hold the rescue pole securely in a vertical position with one end on the bottom of the pool. Participants grab the pole and climb, hand over hand, down the pole to get to the bottom of the pool. Participants should exhale slowly through the nose as they descend.

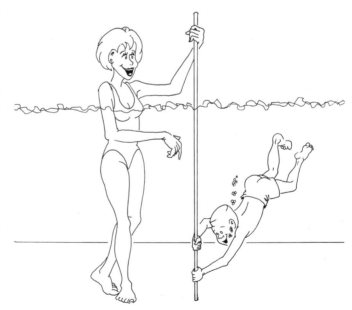

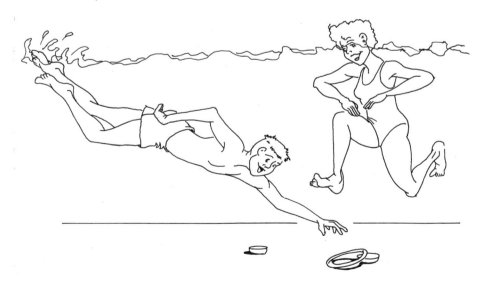

Variation
Fire Pole works in deep water to familiarize swimmers with deeper water. Hold the pole down close to the pool wall and support it from a position on deck. Do not allow more than one participant on the pole at a time. Make this more challenging by placing an object on the bottom within reach of the pole and asking participants to bring it to the surface.

Safety
The pole should be supported by the teacher only. Do not force participants to go all the way to the bottom; they should go only as far as they can. Do not allow hyperventilation.

OBJECT RETRIEVAL

Objectives
Water adjustment; to improve comfort of doing submersion skills without support

Prerequisites
Independent locomotion; submersion

Number of Participants
Limited only by the size of the playing area and availability of equipment

Equipment
Objects that do not float (one per person)

Description
Participants must reach underwater with the hands and retrieve an object off the bottom of the pool.

Variations

- Use the rescue pole to get underwater.
- *Team retrieval:* See variations for Object Retrieval Race listed on page 95 in chapter 5 for ideas on how to set up this game.

Safety

You may assist participants to the bottom by pressing gently on their backs as they attempt to reach for the object. Be sure the participants are aware that you will assist.

CRACK THE WHIP

Objectives

Water adjustment; body control; balance; improved confidence

Prerequisites

Independent locomotion; possibly submersion (if someone goes underwater to move between participants during play)

Number of Participants

Limited only by the size of the playing area

Description

All participants join hands to make a line. The first person in the line leads the group around the pool, twisting and turning. Participants try to follow without letting go of hands. Participants take turns being the leader.

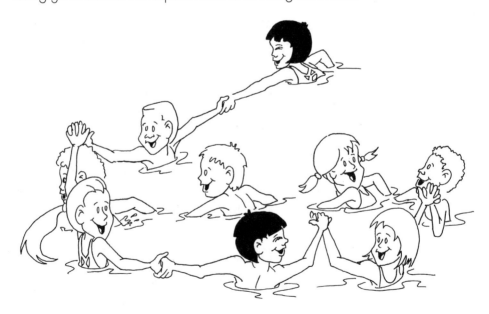

Variation
If participants have submersion skills, have them duck under arms to make the whip more challenging.

Safety
Maintain close supervision. Moving water can cause swimmers to lose their footing.

Stunts and Skills

The skills in this section build on the skills from the previous section, and they are more challenging. Our hope is that participants have become more comfortable in the horizontal position and have enjoyed the process of learning to swim. Although participants can actively participate without total submersion, encourage them to continue to try submersion skills as they practice the horizontal position.

INDEPENDENT KICKING

Objective
Forward progress using a flutter kick

Prerequisites
Independent locomotion; flutter kick while holding onto the side of the pool

Number of Participants
Limited only by the size of the playing area and availability of equipment

Equipment
Kickboard, noodle, or ball (size of a volleyball, soccer ball, or water polo ball) for each participant or pair

Description
Participants grip the object and try to travel forward using a flutter kick. Be sure that they emphasize kicking down with the lower leg.

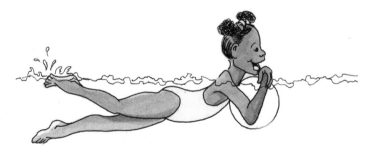

Variation
If you do not have equipment for all participants, use a shuttle relay format and give each team one piece of equipment. Participants travel between boundaries, handing the equipment off to the next person in line.

Safety
Do not allow nonswimmers to kick into deep water while using a handheld object for buoyant support. Be sure that all participants are traveling in the same direction. In the learning stages, you may need to support the kickboard for apprehensive swimmers who cannot control the board themselves. They may experience more success kicking with a ball that can be clutched tightly to the chest.

WHEELBARROW

Objectives
Cooperation; socialization; inclusion; improvement of stroke mechanics

Prerequisites
Independent locomotion; submersion; swimming strokes from chapter 4

Number of Participants
Limited only by the size of the playing area

Description
Pair up participants. Partner A assumes a facedown front float position. Partner B grabs the feet of the partner (as if holding the handle of the wheelbarrow) and walks or jogs, pushing the wheelbarrow across the pool.

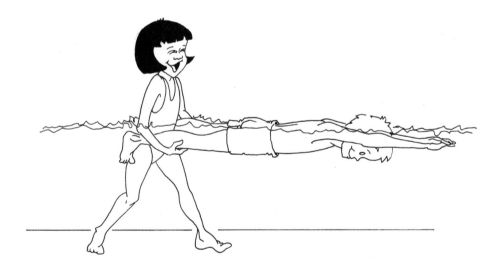

Variations

- Partner A may extend the arms out to the side (shoulders abducted) to create resistance for the partner pushing the wheelbarrow.
- One partner may ride a kickboard while the other pushes him across the pool.
- Do a relay race, with partners changing positions after the first leg of the race.
- Partner A may swim the front crawl or breaststroke.

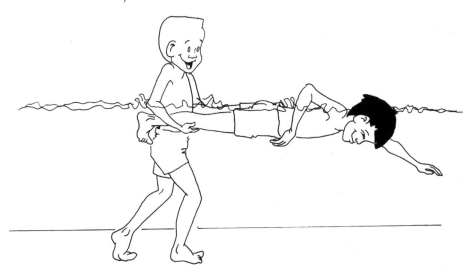

BURN OUT

Objectives
Cooperation; socialization; inclusion; muscular endurance in the upper body

Prerequisites
Submersion; crawl stroke or backstroke

Number of Participants
Limited only by the size of the playing area

Description
Pair up participants. Partner A supports partner B from behind, holding the legs as in the Wheelbarrow (page 126). Partner B swims the crawlstroke as fast as he can and tries to drag partner A forward. As partner B is being pulled forward, he releases the legs of the swimmer, who bursts forward after spinning his wheels from the "burn out."

Variation
The swimmer uses the backstroke.

Safety
Be sure to warm up well before trying to swim hard.

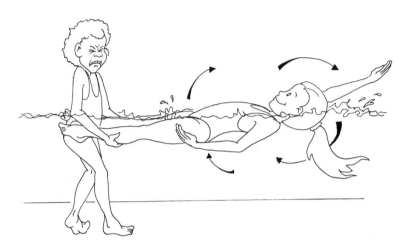

HYDROJETS

Objectives
Unsupported propulsion; streamlining (finding the position of least resistance)

Prerequisites
Independent locomotion; submersion (optional); unsupported front floating

Number of Participants
Limited only by the size of the playing area

Description
Practice pushing from the wall (like a jet taking off) with arms extended in front of the body. Try to glide as far as possible without putting the feet down. Then return to the side using a form of independent locomotion (walk, jog, ski, hop, skip).

Hydrojets can be performed face in or face out, depending on the readiness of the participant. Performing this skill in a faceup position causes the legs to sink more quickly and results in much shorter glides. Better swimmers can practice the skill underwater. This is the lead-up skill for swimming underwater.

Safety
Make sure that participants can get their feet back underneath them to stand up after they perform the skill.

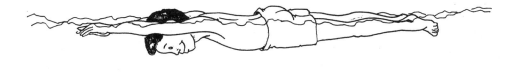

FLIP-FLOPS

Objectives
Rolling over; flutter kick; independent propulsion

Prerequisites
Independent locomotion; flutter kick

Number of Participants
Limited only by the size of the playing area and the availability of equipment

Equipment
Kickboard or ball (size of a soccer ball) for each participant; whistle

Description
This activity should take place in shallow to chest-deep water (deeper with skilled swimmers). Participants kick across the pool on their front or back, using a ball or board for support. Use a whistle to signal. When the whistle blows, participants flip over and continue kicking.

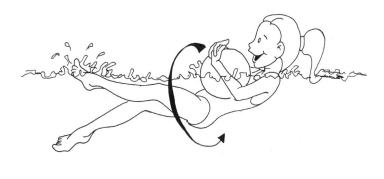

Variations

- *Partner flip-flops:* Partner A walks backward, towing partner B in the front float position. On the count of three, B rolls to his back with the help of A. Have participants put their faces in the water during front kicking. Be sure that signals are no more than 5 seconds apart.

- Use life jackets.

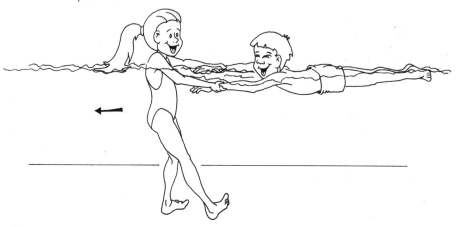

Safety

Do not allow nonswimmers to kick into deep water with their equipment. Make sure all participants are going in the same direction.

PORPOISE DIVES

Objectives

Lead-up for headfirst entry; confidence in underwater skills

Prerequisites

Independent locomotion; submersion; fish flops

Number of Participants

Limited only by the size of the playing area

Description

Participants pretend to be porpoises. Begin in a standing position with arms above the head. Bend the knees and push off the bottom, dive over the surface of the water, and reach for the bottom of the pool. Tuck the head between the arms during the dive. Keep the arms in front of the head until the hands touch the bottom. Push off the bottom with the hands and return to a standing position.

Safety

Be sure that all participants keep their arms over their heads throughout the dive to keep from hitting their heads on the bottom. Have all participants keep their eyes open and travel in the same direction to avoid collisions.

SQUID SWIM

Objective
Improved feel for the water as a force to propel the swimmer, regardless of direction. As the swimmer pushes against the water to go backward, the water pushes back. This skill challenges the swimmer to think differently about locomotion in the water; a lead-up to feet first surface dive.

Prerequisites
Independent locomotion; submersion; lying on the bottom

Number of Participants
Limited only by the size of the playing area

Description
Participants travel feetfirst and facedown on the bottom of the pool. Begin by lying on the bottom. Bend the elbows and bring the hands to rest on the shoulders. Keeping the hands close to the body, slowly bring the arms back to the sides. With palms facing away from the body, forcefully pull the arms (water) over the head as if to clap the hands together above the head. This is the same action the arms make when doing a feetfirst surface dive. Keep the legs together and straight. Continue backward, feetfirst, using the reverse arm pull to travel.

Safety
Do not allow participants to hyperventilate before attempting this skill. Have all participants keep their eyes open and travel in the same direction to avoid collisions.

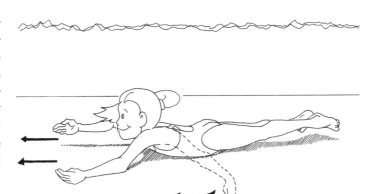

LOG ROLL

Objectives
Swimming independence; rolling over

Prerequisite
Submersion; unsupported floating; hydrojets; flip-flops

Number of Participants
Limited only by the size of the playing area

Description
Push off the wall like a jet and roll over, front to back, in one direction as many times as possible before putting the feet on the bottom. Participants may perform this in a face-in or face-out position. They may use the arms and hands to roll, but some participants will discover that they can do it using only trunk flexion and extension.

Safety
Do not encourage long periods of breath holding. Participants who can do more than three or four log rolls in a row will have a tendency to get dizzy and disoriented. Do not perform this skill in deep water.

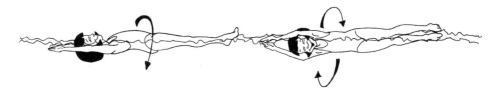

KICKING WAR

Objectives
Cooperation; socialization; inclusion; kicking strength

Prerequisites
Submersion; unsupported floating; independent kicking

Number of Participants
Limited only by the size of the playing area

Description
Partners face each other and grab hands, palm to palm. They assume a prone position with the face in and kick (flutter kick, breaststroke kick) as hard as they can and try to push the other person back.

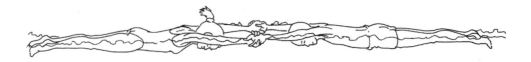

Variation
Use a kickboard between partners.

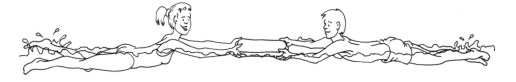

THREAD THE NEEDLE

Objectives
Cooperation; body awareness

Prerequisites
Independent locomotion; submersion; breath control

Number of Participants
Limited only by the size of the playing area

Description
Three partners hold hands to form a small circle. One person is designated the **thread**. She tucks the knees so the legs will rise and then extends the legs across the arms of the other two partners. At the same time, the partners pull the thread through the needle (across the top of the clasped hands and to a position outside the circle).

Safety
The person designated as the thread may submerge and get water up her nose as she is being pulled forward. Remind participants to hum or use nose bubbles.

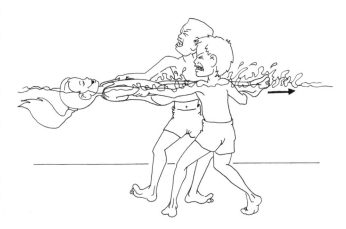

CORKSCREW

Objectives
Body awareness; stroking skills

Prerequisites
Submersion; swimming (front crawl, back crawl); flip-flops

Number of Participants
Limited only by the size of the playing area

Description
Begin by swimming the front crawl (face in or face out). Perform one stroke (right arm) on the front crawl and then roll over from front to back and perform a stroke (left arm) of the back crawl. Continue the front crawl with the right arm and the back crawl with the left arm as you move across the pool. Roll in the same direction each time so that it looks like a corkscrew.

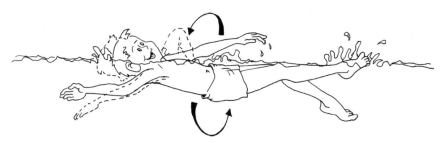

Variations
- Combine strokes to be performed in a corkscrew. For example, do one stroke cycle of front crawl, roll to the side and do two side strokes, roll to the back and do one stroke cycle of backstroke, and continue.
- Perform two breaststrokes, roll to the side for two side strokes, then roll to the back for elementary backstroke or back crawl.

Safety
Watch for dizziness or disorientation. Have participants keep the face out, spot something at the other end of the pool, and swim toward it. Participants should all be moving in the same direction to avoid collisions.

SCULLING

Objectives
Control of body position using only the arms; upper-body strength; treading water

Prerequisite
Floating (independent back float or glide with ears wet)

Description

Sculling is the basic skill used to tread water and to change positions, especially for synchronized swimming. Begin the progression by learning the sculling motion in a standing position in chest-deep water. Position the arms in front of the body at the surface of the water. Turn palms down and bend elbows slightly. Press on the water as if smoothing sand, moving the arms in a figure-eight motion.

Palms turn in slightly as they press in toward the midline of the body and then

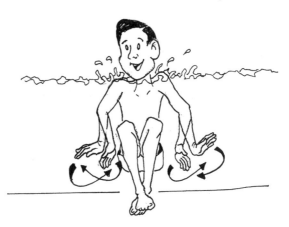

turn out slightly as they press out to the side. If participants are applying enough downward pressure on the water, they should be able to lift the feet off the bottom by bending the knees into the chest and maintain a suspended position by using only the arm power. Once participants have mastered this progression, they are ready to learn the other basic sculling positions.

- *Standard Scull:* Begin on the back, legs extended and straight, toes pointed (this is known as a **back layout position**). Keep the arms extended along the sides and perform the figure eights with the hands close to the hips. Do not kick the legs. Travel headfirst by hyperextending the wrists and pointing the fingertips upward. Press back on the water during the figure eights to travel headfirst.

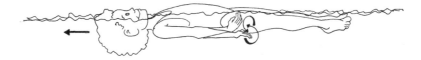

Standard Scull.

- *Snail Scull:* In the same position as in the standard scull, travel feetfirst like a snail by flexing the wrists and pointing the fingers toward the bottom of the pool. Perform the figure eights in this position and pull the water behind and underneath the body, toward the head (if you pull water one direction you will travel in the opposite direction,

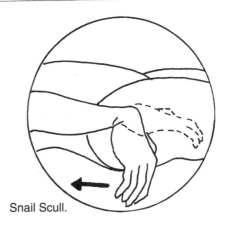

Snail Scull.

according to the principle of action and reaction). Keep the legs straight and the toes pointed and on the surface to decrease the resistance to feetfirst momentum.

- *Torpedo Scull:* This is a more advanced sculling technique and is often difficult to learn. It is very challenging for good swimmers. Begin by using a snail scull to travel feetfirst. Keep the arms underwater. Turn palms away from the body and pull the arms forcefully to a position overhead. Continue sculling with the arms overhead. Wrists are hyperextended so that the fingertips point to the bottom of the pool. Push the water back with the palms to travel feetfirst. Feet and legs must stay at the surface to reduce resistance.

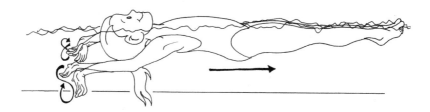

Variations

- Use the standard scull to perform a tuck or tub position.

- Start in a standard scull. Draw the knees toward the chest, keeping only the shins on the surface as the knees come toward the face. The tub is a basic position for some of the deep-water gymnastics skills described next.

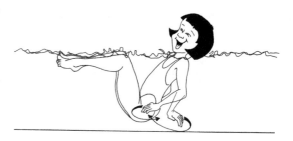

- Tub turn in a circle (scull the water in the opposite direction that you want to turn).

- Tub and extend one leg above the water like a periscope. This position is also known as a *flamingo position.*

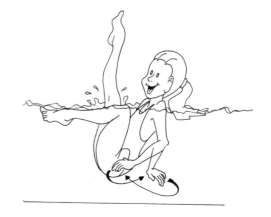

DOWN THE RIVER

Objectives
Relaxation during the back float; controlling body movement in moving water

Prerequisites
Independent locomotion; unsupported floating on back; sculling

Number of Participants
10 to 15 per group

Description
Form a tight circle near a corner in the shallow end of the pool. Have participants grab hands and run around the circle as fast as they can. This creates a whirlpool of fast-moving water. When they have reached peak speed, someone signals and all participants release hands and immediately assume a back floating position. The water crashing into the wall in the corner moves down along the wall, taking the participants *down the river* with it. For safety, teach participants to relax on their backs and turn to get their feet on the surface so they are headed *downstream* in moving water. Once the participants have learned how to *ride the river current,* challenge them to turn and float feetfirst downstream. They can use their sculling skills to accomplish this task.

Safety
Organize the group so that the whirlpool sends them down the river along the shallow-end wall rather than toward the deep water.

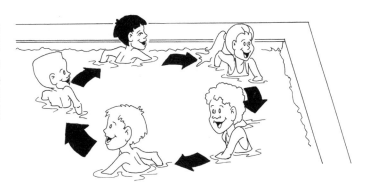

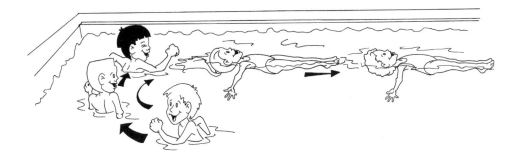

TANDEM SWIM

Objectives
Cooperation; muscular endurance

Prerequisites
Swimming (both partners must be able to swim the same stroke); sculling

Number of Participants
Limited only by the size of the playing area

Description
Partners decide how to hook up so that one person swims half of the stroke while the other person swims the other half. For example, the following are some possibilities:

Front crawl: The lead swimmer hooks his feet at the waist of the trailing swimmer. The trailing swimmer swims faceup and the lead swimmer swims facedown (taking a breath when needed). Both swimmers use arms. The trailing swimmer also uses legs. They try to synchronize the strokes to be more efficient.

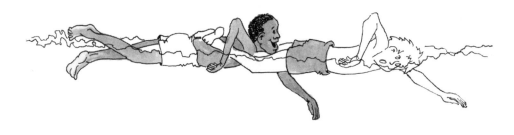

Backstroke: The lead swimmer hooks her feet under the armpits of the trailing swimmer. The lead swimmer uses only the arms. The trailing swimmer uses arms and legs. They try to synchronize the arm strokes to be more efficient.

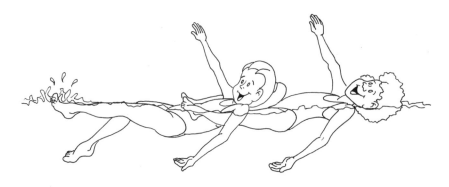

Breaststroke: The lead swimmer hooks her feet at the trailing swimmer's waist. The lead swimmer does only the arm stroke. The trailing swimmer does the whole stroke. They try to synchronize the arm strokes to be more efficient.

Side-by-side swim: Swimmers lie side by side and hook elbows and swim backstroke or elementary backstroke.

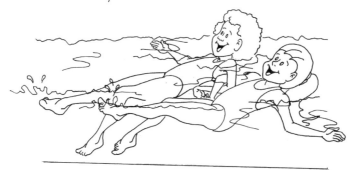

Relay: Swim one leg of the race, and then partners switch places to complete the race.

FLOAT PATTERNS

Objectives
Cooperation; problem solving; comfort in the back float position

Prerequisites
Independent locomotion; supported floating on back; sculling

Number of Participants
Depending on the size of the playing area and the number of participants in a group, as few as 3 and as many as 12

Equipment
None required, but for variety, use whatever is available to enhance the complexity of the float pattern

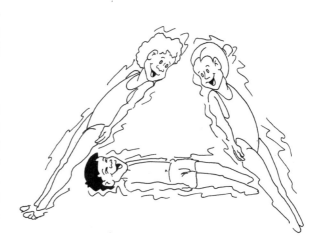

Description
Assign a task and let the members of the group figure out how to accomplish it. For example, groups of three or four form a floating letter. Participants support each other or float to create a letter, number, or float pattern.

Variations

- Give participants a math question and make them form the answer with float patterns.
- Use with the Whistle Stop Stunt Race described later in this chapter.

PLANKING

Objectives
Cooperation; sculling on the back

Prerequisites
Submersion; unsupported floating on back; sculling

Number of Participants
Limited only by the size of the playing area

Description
Partners line up in a back layout position (on back, legs extended straight, toes pointed). The lead swimmer has his feet on or near the shoulders of the trail swimmer. The trail swimmer reaches back and grabs the lead swimmer's ankles. He then submerges and pulls the lead swimmer over the top of him in an effort to change places with the lead swimmer.

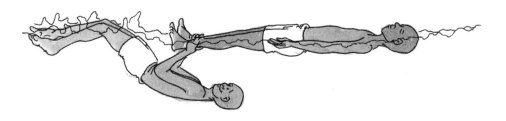

STUFF IT

Objectives
Cooperation; fun; socialization

Prerequisite
Independent locomotion

Number of Participants
Five per group; number of groups limited only by the size of the playing area

Equipment
One latex swim cap per group (have extra caps in case one breaks)

Description

The object of the stunt is to get the latex swim cap big enough to stuff one member of the team into it. Four members of the team form a small circle and hold the cap at the edges with their fingertips.

They enlarge the cap by forcing it up and down underwater against the weight of the water (a latex cap gets very large). The fifth member of the team (the stuffee) is positioned just behind two members of the group with one hand on each member's shoulder. When the cap is big enough for the stuffee, she quickly jumps over the group's arms and lowers herself into the cap. This must be timed with the group pulling the cap up from underwater, or it will not work. The stuffers then pull the cap up around the neck of the stuffee and carry her to the finish line. (This is modified slightly from the *stuff it* contest played by advanced competitive swimmers. In the competitive version the stuffee must take a breath and go completely inside the cap and then is dragged across the pool to the finish line. This makes *stuff it* a breath-holding contest, and therefore it is not a safe option.)

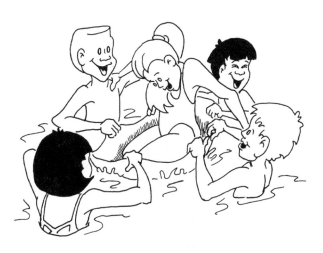

WATER GYMNASTICS

Objectives

Advanced water skills; breath control; confidence; feeling of accomplishment (These skills are much easier to learn if the participant has tried some gymnastics on a floor mat.)

Prerequisites

Independent locomotion; submersion

Description

Teach the following skills as you would in a land gymnastics class: handstand, walk on hands, front walkover (start as in a handstand and walk the feet forward one at a time to contact the water), standing front flip, and back handspring.

Variations

- Begin front flips and back handsprings in the horizontal (floating) position. These are lead-up skills for the pike surface dive and front flip turns.

- *Front flip in a circle:* Make a circle and grab hands. On the signal all participants try a front flip. This keeps everyone from holding their noses. For an added challenge, see who can do two in a row without breaking the links of hands.

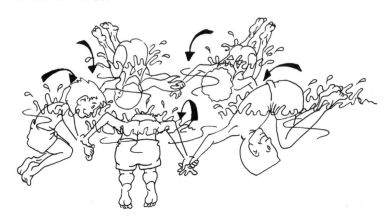

- *Kickboard gymnastics:* Sit on a kickboard, trapping it behind the knees, and try a front flip and a back flip. Try a handstand on the kickboard. For safety reasons, be sure that participants have plenty of room in case their boards get away from them.

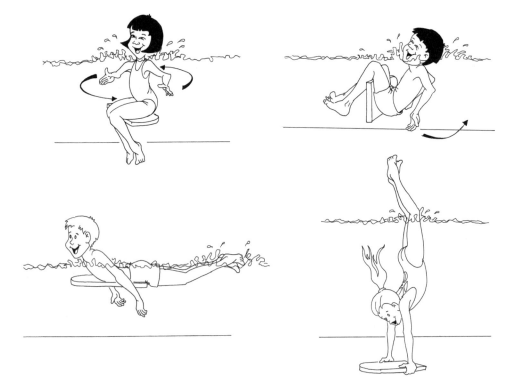

Safety

Spot participants or teach spotting techniques to partners. Make sure that all participants are practicing in the same direction. Keep eyes open. Because participants will be inverted (upside down) during the skills, they need to blow the air out using nose bubbles.

PARTNER HANDSTANDS

Objectives

Cooperation; learning to think upside down; body control

Prerequisites

Independent locomotion; submersion; handstands

Number of Participants

Limited only by the size of the playing area

Description

Partners face each other. One person performs a handstand. Then the other person does a handstand, and the two partners try to place the bottoms of their feet together above the water.

Safety

Partners should have a signal that means *come down.* Eyes should be open to avoid collisions. A third person can spot the pair during this stunt.

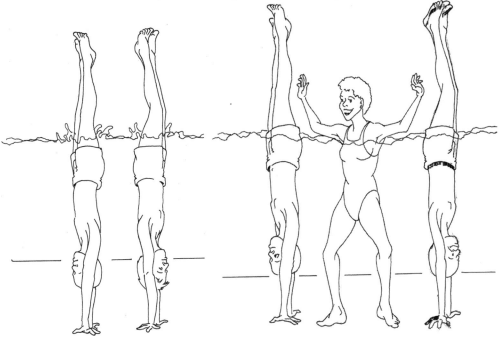

LEAPFROG

Objectives
Breath control; cooperation

Prerequisites
Independent locomotion; submersion; sitting on the bottom

Number of Participants
Limited only by the size of the playing area

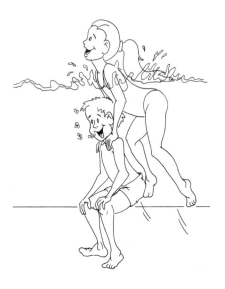

Description
Partners stand facing the same direction, one in front of the other. The partner behind places her hands on the lead partner's shoulders and prepares to jump over him. The partner in front takes a deep breath and squats down on the bottom. The partner behind leaps over, and leapfrog continues with partners taking turns.

Variation
More advanced swimmers can somersault over the front partner. Place hands on the shoulders of the person in front. Push off forward and roll over the top of the partner.

Safety
Make sure participants have their eyes open and stay in control to keep from landing on the partner in front.

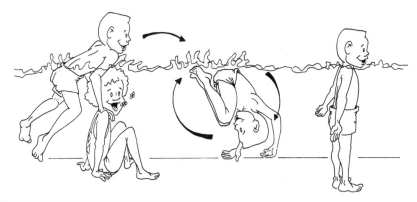

DEEP-WATER GYMNASTICS

Objectives
Deep-water skills, body control using upper-body strength, body awareness

Prerequisites
Submersion; swimming; sculling; shallow-water gymnastics skills (handstands, front flips from a front float position, back handsprings from a back float position); standard scull and tub positions

Number of Participants

Limited only by the size of the playing area

Description

Water gymnastics is a generic term used here to denote synchronized swimming skills. Males are more likely to try "water gymnastics" than "synchronized swimming," which is the reason for the terminology. Here are some deep-water gymnastics skills.

Pike surface dive: Begin in a front float position and pretend to do a handstand. Draw the arms down to the sides. At the same time, drop the head below the hips by bending at the waist. Turn the palms away from the body and pull the arms in a backward circle to a position over the head. This will help raise the legs out of the water. Reach for the bottom. The weight of the legs above the water will force you underwater.

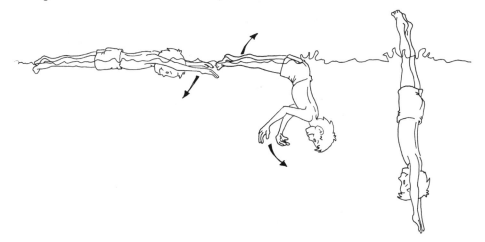

Kip: Begin in a back layout position. Perform the first half of a somersault so that the toes are pointed at the sky and you are upside down. Extend the legs straight up and drop underwater in a vertical position.

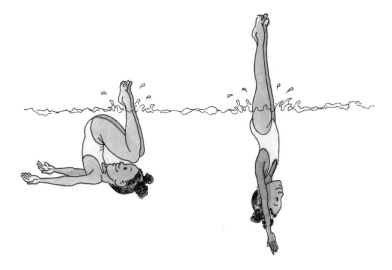

Front somersault: Begin in a tub position. Tuck the chin tightly into the chest and pull the arms hard in a backward circle. Continue circling backward to return to the starting position with the face out. This skill can also be performed from a front float position. Begin as if to do a

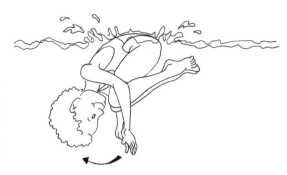

pike surface dive. Instead of reaching for the bottom, keep the head tucked toward the legs and continue pulling backward. Complete the somersault in a back float position or continue to pull around to the starting position.

Back tuck somersault: Begin in a back layout position. Pull slowly into a tight tub position. Pull the arms in a forward circular motion to a position behind the head. Continue pulling to return to the starting tub position and complete the somersault by extending to the back layout.

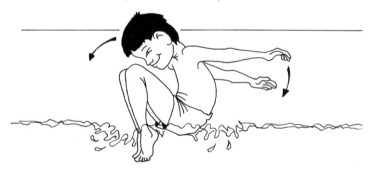

Oyster: Begin in a standard scull (back layout) position, with arms extended along the sides. Turn the palms down and pull the arms forcefully in a circular motion to a position behind the head. At the same time pike hard at the hips to get the legs out of the water. Try to close the oyster by touching the hands to the legs. Sink underwater in this position.

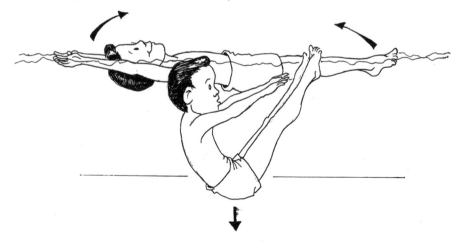

Back dolphin: Begin in a back layout position. Perform as a back handspring in shallow-water gymnastics. Arch the back and look toward the bottom. Continue pulling the arms in a forward circular motion to return to the back layout position. Try to keep the legs straight and the toes pointed.

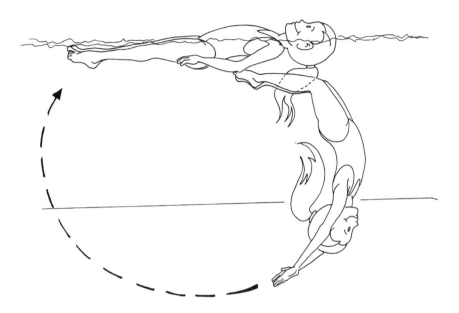

Safety
The minimum water depth required for these skills is 6 feet (about 2 meters) so the participant does not hit the bottom of the pool while performing the skill.

CHAIN DOLPHIN

Objectives
Deep-water skills; breath control; cooperation; body awareness

Prerequisites
Submersion; swimming; sculling; back dolphin

Number of Participants
Limited only by the size of the playing area

Description
In water that is at least 7 feet (a little over 2 meters) deep, partners line up in a back layout. The lead swimmer hooks her feet at the trailing swimmer's neck. The lead swimmer arches her back to go underwater in a back dolphin. The trailing swimmer propels through the chain dolphin by sculling headfirst. Both swimmers use the arms to get the chain around in the back dolphin position. When the lead swimmer surfaces she continues to scull headfirst until the trailing swimmer surfaces.

Safety
Partners should have a signal to break the chain if one is uncomfortable. Do not allow the swimmers to hyperventilate.

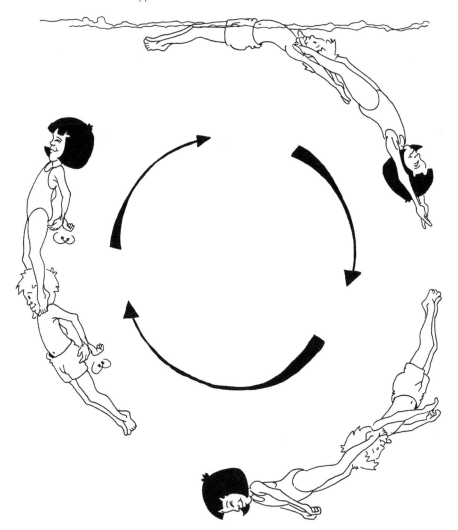

Swimming Games

Swimming games are designed for participants who are very comfortable with submersion skills and can make forward progress with multiple stroke patterns. Participants should be able to swim at least two lengths of the pool and to jump into deep water and tread for at least two minutes. However, many of these games can be adapted so that nonswimmers remain in standing-depth water and advanced participants play the game in the deep end. In addition, you may discover some of your own adaptations to use when a swimmer pairs with a nonswimmer.

FOLLOW THE LEADER

Objectives
Socialization; skill challenge; confidence

Prerequisites
Floating; swimming; sculling; individual stunts (submersion is optional depending on the skill of the group)

Number of Participants
Limited only by the size of the playing area

Description
Designate a leader. The leader travels around the pool performing skills and stunts. Each member of the group tries the skill or stunt. Each participant takes a turn at being leader.

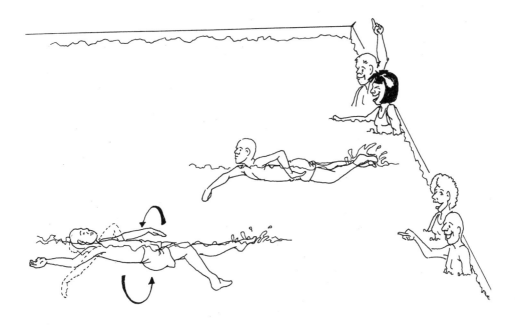

Variation
Use partner stunts.

WHISTLE STOP STUNT RACE

Objectives
Skill execution; confidence; socialization

Prerequisites
Submersion; swimming; sculling; partner stunts and skills from chapter 5; water gymnastics stunts

Number of Participants
Limited only by the size of the playing area

Description
Swimmers race a certain distance using a predetermined method of swimming. On the whistle, participants must stop, complete a stunt (front flip, back flip, handstand, kip, log roll, bob, tub turn, and the like), and then complete the distance. The loser sits out one race and then joins for the next series.

Variations
- Use partner stunts.
- Use a team of three or four. One team goes at a time. Each team forms a float pattern or letter. Teams are timed for the whistle stop stunt, and the winning team is the team with the fastest time.

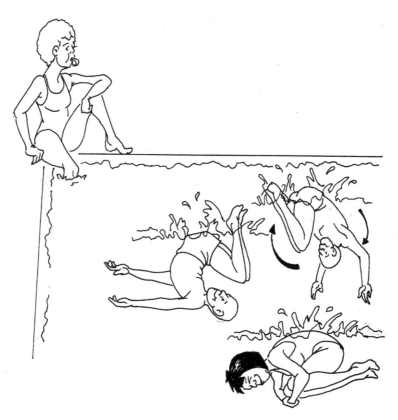

AQUA MAN RELAY

Objectives
Breath control; lead-up for headfirst entry

Prerequisites
Independent locomotion; submersion; porpoise dive

Number of Participants
Two or more equal teams of four to six players

Description
Divide the teams as for a shuttle relay. On the signal, the first person porpoise dives across the pool. He may not swim or take any walking steps between porpoise dives.

Safety
Participants must keep their eyes open to avoid collisions.

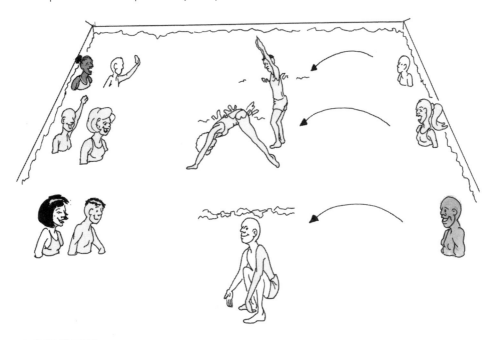

BASEBALL

Objectives
Socialization; cooperation; eye-hand coordination; throwing

Prerequisites
Independent locomotion; swimming skills to play in deep water (outfielder)

Number of Participants
At least 6 per team (9 to 11 per team preferred)

Equipment
Wiffle ball and plastic bat, rubber bases or traffic cones (pylons)

Description
Use standard baseball rules. Adapt rules for age and skill of the participants. If there are swimmers and nonswimmers in the group, select teams so that each has an equal number of nonswimmers for the shallow-water positions. Organize the bases in the shallow area. Deep water is the outfield.

Variations
- Let participants use any method of locomotion to reach the base.
- Set the bases closer together for children.
- Let participants have more than three strikes.
- Let older participants have only one pitch.
- Let participants run either direction around the bases but continue in the original direction chosen.

Safety
If possible, keep the safety line in place. Swimmers can swim under it to field the ball. It will keep nonswimmers from slipping into deeper water.

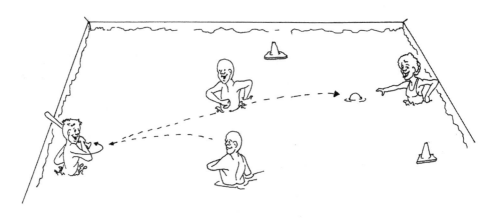

RAG TAG

Objectives
Confidence; socialization

Prerequisites
Independent locomotion; submersion; swimming

Number of Participants
Limited only by the size of the playing area

Equipment
A soft rag tied into a ball, or a foam ball the size of a baseball

Description
One person is designated as It. It tags other participants by hitting them with the rag. Anyone hit with the rag becomes It. Participants may duck under or swim under the water to avoid being tagged. It may tag or throw the ball.

Variations
- *Partner Rag Tag:* A swimmer and nonswimmer may play It as partners and pass the rag back and forth from shallow to deep.
- *Team Rag Tag:* One team is It and they are allowed to pass the ball to each other in order to tag or hit a participant on the other team. When tagged, participants must stop in place, tread, swim, float, or stand and wait until someone on their team touches them to put them back into play. Be sure to give each team equal time to be It.

Safety
If swimmers and nonswimmers are playing together, keep the safety line in place. All play must remain in the water. A rag thrown out of the pool should be retrieved by the teacher and thrown back to It.

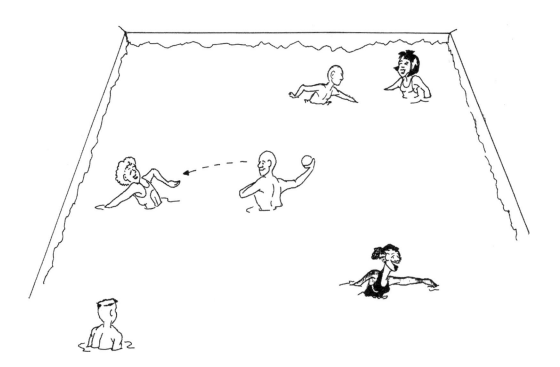

FIN TAG

Objectives
Cardiorespiratory endurance; kick strength; surface diving

Prerequisites
Submersion; swimming; treading water; surface diving

Number of Participants
Limited only by the size of the deep-water area and number of fins

Equipment
One pair of fins per participant

Description
Divide the group into two teams of equal numbers. The object of the game is to see which team can pull more fins off the opposing team in the time allotted. Players let the pulled fins float in the water. Participants who lose both fins go to the side but can reenter the game if someone retrieves one or both of the fins.

Safety
Do not allow participants to make physical contact with players except by touching fins.

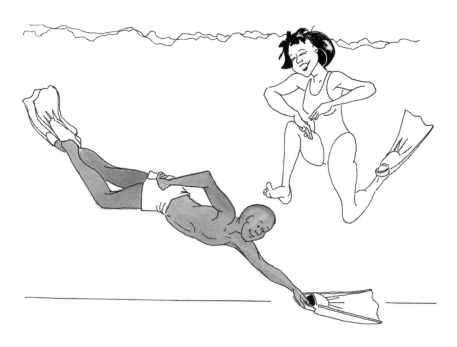

MEDLEY RELAY

Objective
Determined by the skills chosen for locomotion

Prerequisite
Swimming

Number of Participants
Two or more equal teams of four to six players

Description
Use a shuttle relay formation. Each member of the team is given a different stroke to swim across the pool (for example, front crawl, back crawl, elementary backstroke, sidestroke, breaststroke, butterfly, or a stroke variation). On the signal, the first member completes the distance and tags the second person, who travels back across the pool. The relay continues until all members of the team have completed their leg of the race.

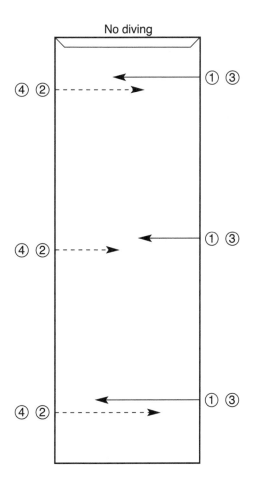

Variations

- Have all swimmers swim the same stroke.
- Use forms of the corkscrew for locomotion.
- Swim with kickboard stunts.
- Use the shuttle relay format. This relay starts in the water. Each team has a dry towel or a newspaper. Each member of the team swims his leg of the relay without getting the towel or newspaper wet. The winner is the team with the fastest time and the driest towel or newspaper.
- See additional variations in chapter 5, such as Partner Relay.

Safety
If starting from the deck, do not allow dive entries into water less than 9 feet (about 3 meters) deep.

BALL RELAY

Objective
Lead-up for water polo

Prerequisite
Swimming front crawl with the head up

Number of Participants
Two or more even teams of four to six players

Equipment
One ball per team, all the same size

Description
Divide the teams as for a shuttle relay. On the signal, the first person swims the ball across the pool using the front crawl. The ball is kept moving in front of the swimmer by the action of the arm stroke as the swimmer's arm reaches forward for the next stroke (as in water polo). She gives the ball to the second team member, and the relay continues until all members of the team have completed their leg of the race.

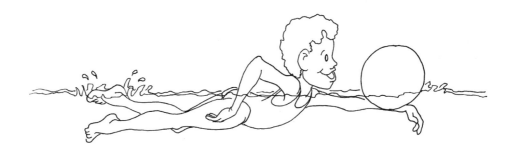

Variations
- Organize the teams in a single-file line. Each member of the team swims the distance and shoots for a goal. Have a team member catch the ball or use chairs to mark the goal. Points are awarded for the most goals in the shortest amount of time.
- Hold the ball between the knees. Swim on the front or back. A ball that pops out must be retrieved.
- Use the shuttle relay format. Each team has a spoon with a Ping-Pong ball on it. The swimmer swims the front crawl carrying the spoon in her mouth, then hands it off to the next person in the relay.

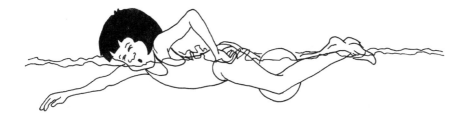

TANDEM RELAY

Objectives
Determined by skills chosen for locomotion; interval training

Prerequisite
Swimming (both partners must be able to swim the same stroke)

Number of Participants
Two or more teams of four, six, or eight players

Description
All members of the team are positioned on the same end of the pool. Each team member has a partner. Each pair completes two legs of the race using a predetermined partner swim. (See Individual and Partner Stunts in chapter 5.) If the race involves a partner stunt where one person leads, partners trade places after the first leg of the race. The relay continues until all pairs have completed their legs of the race. The winning team is the team who completes all legs of the race the fastest.

Safety
If the relay begins on the deck, do not allow headfirst entries (dives) in water that is less than 9 feet (about 3 meters) deep. Do not allow swimmers to help each other out of the water.

SWIM THE WAVES

Objectives
Socialization; swimming in moving water; muscular endurance in the chest and upper-back muscles; core stability

Prerequisites
Submersion; swimming; treading water

Number of Participants
Large groups, twenty or more per group

Equipment
One kickboard per participant

Description
Participants, each with a kickboard, form two lines in the deep water, facing each other about 10 feet apart. Participants use the broad side of the kickboard to make a gauntlet of waves by alternately pushing and pulling the board through the surface of the water. One swimmer tries to swim through the waves between the two lines. Take turns letting all swimmers challenge the waves.

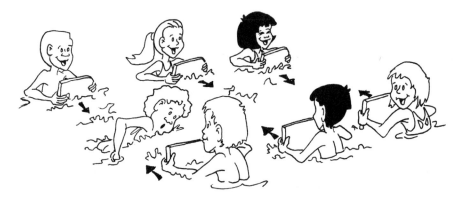

Variation
To practice throwing rescues, have each participant take a turn standing on the deck and throwing a heaving jug, heaving line, or ring buoy into the wave machine to pull a swimmer through the waves to safety. The swimmer in the water may kick to assist the rescue.

Safety
Swimmers should tread water and exit the waves if they cannot swim from one end to the other.

LIFE JACKET WATER POLO

Objectives
Independence in deep water; eye–hand coordination; cardiorespiratory endurance; interval training

Prerequisites
Ability to control body position while wearing a life jacket; swim and return to the side in a life jacket

Number of Participants
Two teams of equal numbers, limited only by the size of the playing area

Equipment
Some form of identification to separate the teams (colored latex caps are not too expensive—have the captains flip a coin to see who has to wear the caps);

life jackets for each participant; a water polo ball, or use a small beach ball to keep play unpredictable; goals, or equipment to designate goals (traffic cones [pylons] work pretty well)

Description

Use standard water polo rules (for rules and regulations visit www.usawaterpolo. com). To begin play, the referee tosses the ball up between two teams who try to retrieve it and advance it to score a goal. One point is awarded for each goal. After a goal, the ball is put in play as in the beginning of the game. Players must pass the ball with one hand to score. Goals can be scored only if attempted from behind the goal line. Adapt the rules to fit the age and skill of the group. Examples of rule adaptations include the following: All players may throw with both hands, players may rest on the sideline for 10 to 30 seconds, and there must be three passes before a goal can be scored.

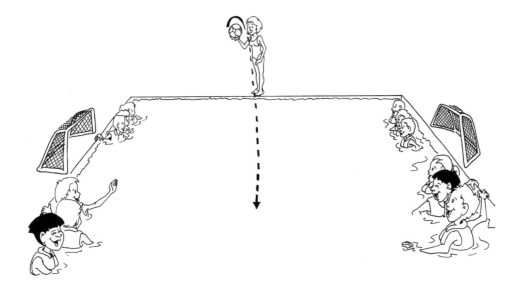

Variations

- *Play without life jackets:* For intervals, divide each team in half. One group plays two minutes while the other group hangs on the wall. At the signal, groups alternate positions. This allows hard, continuous interval play.

- *Nonswimmers wear life jackets, swimmers do not:* A nonswimmer must make the goal. Swimmers play water polo across the deep end of the pool. Nonswimmers play in chest-deep water. Nonswimmers must hit the ball and pass as in volleyball. The ball can be hit any number of times and then may be thrown for a goal.

- If the pool slopes from shallow to deep, water polo can be played using the length of the pool. Divide the teams evenly, with the same number of swimmers and nonswimmers on each team. Keep the safety line in place. Swimmers, both offensive and defensive, may not pass the safety line to make plays in the shallow end. Nonswimmers, both offensive and defensive, carry on the game in the shallow half of the pool. Playing the length of the pool usually increases the playing area, but this method is more challenging and fun for both groups.

- Limit the number of in-water players and rotate every few minutes.
- Limit the number of in-water players, but allow other members of the team to keep the ball in play from poolside. Players must sit at the edge of the pool. They may not stand or chase the ball on deck. Any ball that goes behind a deck player is out of bounds.
- *Volleyball variation:* Players must either hit the ball or use a two-handed overhead pass to advance it.

Safety
If a standard water polo ball is used, players must wear headgear to protect the ears from injury by a hard-thrown ball. A beach ball is a good alternative because it does not hurt if thrown hard, it takes funny spins in the air because of its size and weight, and it keeps the game challenging, interesting, and fun.

UNDERWATER HOCKEY

Objectives
Confidence; underwater swimming; socialization

Prerequisites
Independent locomotion; submersion; underwater swimming; porpoise dive; treading water

Number of Participants
Two teams, numbers limited only by the size of the playing area

Equipment
One hockey puck, a hockey stick and glove for each player, goals at each end of the playing area. A rubber diving ring is a good substitute for a hockey puck. Sticks can be made from wood and should be 11 inches (28 centimeters) long. Drill a hole through the handle of the stick and attach a wrist strap of some kind to keep the stick from floating away if it is released during play. Use traffic cones (pylons) to mark the goals on the bottom of the pool.

Description
Use standard underwater hockey rules (www.underwater-society.org). One member from each team faces off over the puck to begin the game. Players must leave the puck on the bottom of the pool when they return to the surface for air.

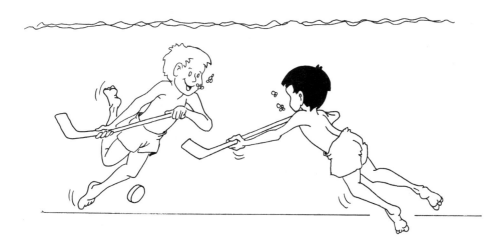

Variation
Increase the playing area and allow participants to wear masks, fins, and snorkels.

Safety
Caution players against hyperventilation. Players should wear a garden glove or an inexpensive work glove with the knuckle area covered with solidified hot glue to protect the knuckles during play. (To apply, put gloves on hands and spread warmed hot glue over the knuckles. Let dry to solidify.)

BIG SPLASH CONTEST

Objective
Approach to a spring dive

Prerequisites
Independent locomotion; submersion; swimming; treading water

Equipment
1-meter diving board, diving scorecards

Description
The water under the diving board should be at least 11.5 feet (3.5 meters) deep. Select three people to serve as judges. Participants make three jumps from the board, using a feetfirst entry. Each jump is awarded a score by the judges. Judges use a scale from 1 to 10, and they award scores according to the height and width of the splash. The person who accumulates the most total points in three jumps is the winner. If two participants tie, they may have a splash-off, which consists of one final attempt.

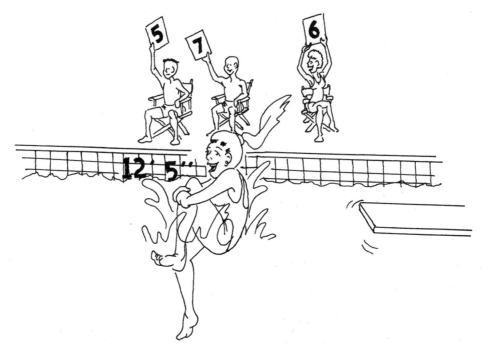

Variation

Throw a ball to the contestant at the height of the jump. Points are awarded only if the contestant catches the ball.

Safety

Standard diving board rules apply. Do not use a board or platform higher than 1 meter. Do not allow swimmers to help each other out of the water.

Fitness Swimming

Swimming is an excellent form of exercise. It benefits the cardiovascular and musculoskeletal systems and maintains flexibility, especially in the shoulder joints. It is also a great activity to use for cross-training, meaning that you can supplement your aqua basics and sport aqua workouts with some fitness swimming for cardiorespiratory endurance or for interval training. Many books describe how to set up interval training in swimming, so we will not be addressing it here. Just remember the parts of the interval set and you will be able to use your knowledge and creativity to apply it to these fitness swimming activities (see Interval Training on page 9).

Unless you have a small group or a very large pool (25 to 40 lanes), you will not have the luxury of assigning each participant a lane. Fun laps, in which many participants share a lane and swim whatever strokes they like, help organize the class so that continuous lap swimming can occur without people encountering traffic jams or waiting in line for a turn. Participants who feel comfortable in a life jacket may participate in

Table 6.1 Yard and Meter Conversion

Distance	Meters	Yards
1 lap	50	50
2 laps	100	100
8 laps	400 (1/4 mile)	400
9 laps	450	450 (1/4 mile)**
16 laps	800 (1/2 mile)	800
18 laps	900	900 (1/2 mile)**
32 laps	1,600 (1 mile)*	1,600
36 laps	1,800	1,800 (1 mile)**

* 1,609.35 meters = 1 mile

** 1,760 yards = 1 mile

lap swims as well. The objective of the fun laps is to work on swimming endurance. Because training improvements are specific, in order to build cardiorespiratory endurance for swimming, you must swim the aerobic set. These fun laps are a method of building swimming endurance one length of the pool at a time. See table 6.1 for a conversion of numbers of laps to meters and yards.

Here are some methods of organizing fun laps to ensure that swimmers don't get in each other's way and to keep fitness swimming interesting.

CATCH-UP SWIM

Description

This is the easiest progression for continuous lap swimming because swimmers take a rest at each wall. It allows the swimmer to have the entire lane to navigate. Divide the class equally among the lanes. Within each lane, have participants organize themselves according to speed, with the fastest swimmer being the leader. On a signal, send the lead swimmer off. Send each succeeding swimmer off at five-second intervals. When the lead swimmer reaches the end wall, he waits until all swimmers in his lane have completed the length, then he starts a new length. Swimmers must maintain the same order so that they all receive about the same amount of rest on the wall.

Variations

- Have leader change strokes at each wall.
- Use kickboard lengths.
- Perform partner swims.

ZIGZAG SWIM

Description
This is a Follow the Leader swim. Organize the class with faster swimmers first. Send the first swimmer down the lane. Send the next swimmers every 10 seconds. When the lead swimmer reaches the end wall, he swims back in the next lane. After the lead swimmer has completed all laps, he gets out of the pool and walks to the start to begin the new zigzag. Swimmers may stop at each end wall to rest or let another swimmer pass. However, zigzags are more challenging and effective if done continuously.

Variations
- Have leaders change stroke method for each length.
- Select a new leader for each round.
- Perform partner swims.
- Have swimmers do a stunt (water gymnastics) in the middle of each length.

Safety
Do not allow swimmers to help each other out of the water.

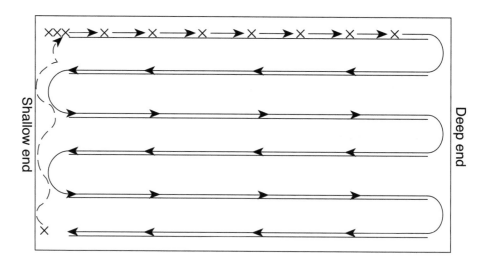

FOUR CORNERS

Description
Swim around the pool next to the wall. Jog across the shallow end to finish the lap.

Variation
Use different forms of locomotion to travel across the shallow end each time.

CIRCLES AROUND THE POOL

Description
Same as Four Corners, but keep a big circle and everyone must swim, not walk, in the shallow water. Swimmers must swim at about the same pace.

Variations
- Swim a circle within a circle. Less conditioned swimmers can swim the outside circle so that they have access to the wall.
- Have circles go in opposite directions.
- Have swimmers swim a circle in deep water and nonswimmers run a circle in shallow water.
- Swim a figure eight and cross each other's paths as you swim the figure.

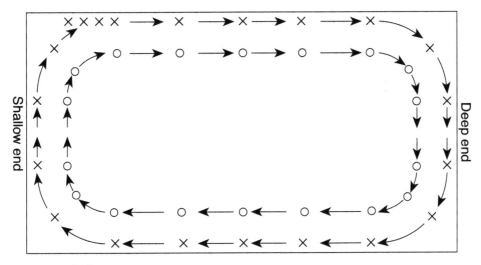

O = Swimmers
X = Nonswimmers

CIRCLES IN THE LANE

Description
This is also known as circle swimming. Most facilities encourage circle swimming to accommodate more than one swimmer per lane. Swimmers swim down on one side of the lane and back on the other in a counter-clockwise direction. Teach students correct lap swimming etiquette. Create or find a lane where swimmers can swim at a similar speed or a similar workout. For example, swimmers who want to do stroke drills with buoys or kickboards could be in the same lane and those who want to do continuous swims could swim together in another lane.
If a swimmer needs to pass another swimmer in the same lane, the passing

swimmer signals by touching the foot of the swimmer in the lead. The lead swimmer stops at the nearest wall and lets the other swimmer go in front, then gives the new lead swimmer a 5- to 10-second head start before continuing down the lane.

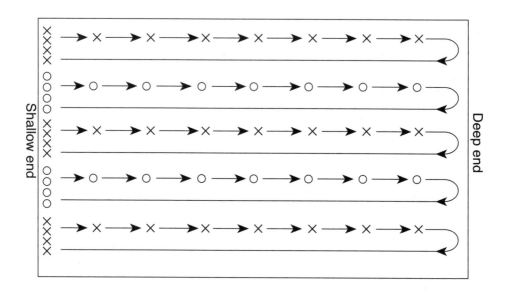

SWIM ACROSS THE ENGLISH CHANNEL

Description

This fitness challenge can be used to challenge swimmers to accomplish more each day. Swimmers may swim any stroke in any fashion (exception: they may not use fins). They may change strokes at any time. Measure the distance of your pool for different "fun laps" described in the previous section.

Give the participants a minimum of one day in three to work toward completion of the English Channel swim. This means that every third day is devoted to continuous swim training for this fitness challenge. For cardiorespiratory endurance fitness benefits, they will need a minimum of 20 minutes of continuous effort or two bouts of 10 minutes each after they have completed the warm-up. The goal distance depends on the swimming skill. An attainable goal for good swimmers is swimming a continuous mile; for less conditioned swimmers, a half-mile is an attainable goal.

Nonswimmers may participate in the shallow end using water running. Individuals who water run should try to cover a half-mile for their fitness challenge.

Place a posterboard in the pool area. It should have a grid for recording distance. Each square on the grid should equal a certain distance covered (e.g., quarter-mile, half-mile, 5 laps, 10 laps, and so on). Those who cannot complete the distance represented by the square in a single day should pencil the completed distance in the square. When the swimmer has completed the total distance, the square can be colored in. For younger participants, use the smaller increments to improve the chances of success. (Example: Determine the average number of laps that the slowest person can complete in 15 minutes. Set the grid up in multiples of this distance.) Give awards for each method of travel.

Variation
Use a local popular body of water instead of the English Channel.

Fitness Challenge Record Grid

Starting date _____   Ending date _____

Simon Mendoza											
Jessica Elder											
Latasha Johnson											
Kevin Tohei											

Each square is worth 5 laps.

MINI-TRIATHLON/BIATHLON

Description
Biathlon and triathlon events are set up the same way. The triathlon event involves swimming, water running, and land running. The biathlon event can be a water run/swim or a swim/land run.

Begin by selecting an appropriate distance for the class or group. For example, swim a quarter-mile, run 100 meters in the pool, and run 400 meters on a track. The more advanced the class, the longer the distances. Measure the distance across the shallow end of the pool to determine how many trips it takes to run the distance you have selected. All participants must run in the same relative depth of water (example: chest deep) to be fair. You can run the event in one day or over a period of three days. Organize the biathlon in the same manner.

Variation

Place a time limit (10 minutes, minimum) on each event and total the number of yards or meters that each participant covers in that period of time. In this way you can select the amount of time you want to spend doing the event in class. You can also select appropriate time limits for each different skill or fitness group represented in your class.

For example, you could have a mini-Tinman triathlon with a 10-minute limit per event and a mini-Ironman triathlon with a 15-minute limit on each event. This allows you to give fitness awards in more categories. You can give awards for best in each single event and for overall winners. If you use these events in a pretest or posttest manner, you can give awards for most improved in each event and overall.

appendix a

Equipment for Water Fun and Safety

Following are descriptions of some of the aquatic equipment you might use in your program, with ideas for how to use them and cautions for their use.

earplugs—These are usually used to reduce the chance of ear infection. People wearing earplugs may find it difficult to hear, and it can be dangerous to use them in depths greater than 6 feet (about 2 meters) underwater because water pressure forces the earplug deeper into the air space of the ear.

fins—Designed to increase the propulsive effect of the kick, fins may be used by weak swimmers to experience better body position or faster swimming. They also can be used as an equalizer in a game or activity situation, or for fitness swimming to improve kick strength and endurance and ankle flexibility.

flotation devices—This term refers to inner tubes and all wearable devices that are not U.S. Coast Guard approved. Each design differs in the amount of buoyancy it provides. Most are designed to assist a learner in maintaining a good body position for learning strokes. Restrict use of flotation devices to shallow water only. Inner tubes may be used in deep water for game activities by good swimmers only.

goggles—Goggles create an air space in front of the eye that protects the eyes from water and increases visibility underwater. They may also decrease apprehension of facial submersion and give the swimmer better awareness of body position in the water. They are dangerous if used when diving from a height, such as a springboard, or if used in depths of more than 4 feet (about 1 meter) because the swimmer has no way to decrease the pressure caused by the water. Goggles may cause damage to the soft tissues around the eyes.

kickboard—A kickboard is designed to float and is used primarily for practicing kicking skills. It can be held in many different positions. It should not be used by weak swimmers in deep water. If used other than for the intended purpose (as in skills described earlier in this book), be sure students can keep the board from rocketing back to the surface and hitting other swimmers.

life jacket—This is a personal flotation device (PFD) designed to be attached and worn by the user. It should be U.S. Coast Guard approved and fit snugly. Though life jackets are the safest choice for nonswimmers who wish to venture into deep water, practice in shallow water is recommended before experimenting in the deep water.

mask—Designed to cover the eyes and nose, a mask is normally used for skin and scuba diving. It increases underwater visibility and allows the swimmer to dive deeper than with goggles because the pressure inside the mask can be equalized by exhaling gently through the nose. A mask may be dangerous if used without supervision; it could fill with water and slip down to cover the mouth and nose. Masks are useful for playing underwater hockey.

noodle—Initially designed as play equipment, these flexible foam tubes now have many uses, from riding to supported kicking to team games. The noodle is rapidly becoming a common poolside amenity. It should not be used in deep water by nonswimmers.

noseplugs—Noseplugs, which keep water out of the nose, are not recommended for learning to swim because they encourage breath holding rather than air exchange. They are more appropriately used for more advanced skills such as synchronized swimming skills, where the swimmer is inverted (upside down). Noseplugs increase breath-holding time because the swimmer does not have to exhale to keep water out of the nose during inverted skills. They would be useful for the water gymnastics skills described in chapter 6.

pull buoy—Usually made of closed cell foam, a pull buoy is designed to be worn between the legs (somewhere between the knees and crotch) to isolate the arms for stroke drills. They are often difficult to use with beginners, who may feel insecure when the legs float too high and they are not sure how to put their feet back on the bottom. Do not allow nonswimmers to use pull buoys as the only means of support in deep water.

rescue equipment—Standard rescue equipment at most pools includes an aluminum reaching pole and a ring buoy. Lifeguards have rescue tubes available that can be used for referee support in the deep end for deep-water games. Other rescue equipment should not be used except in an emergency. If a throwing device is not available, make your own (known as a *heaving jug*) using a 1/4- to 1/2-inch (25 millimeters) nylon rope (25 to 45 feet [about 8 to 14 meters] long) and a heavy plastic container (laundry detergent bottle works well) with the lid. Attach the rope to the handle of the bottle. Fill the bottle with enough water so it is heavy enough to throw accurately. Replace the lid tightly. For more information on basic water rescues, contact your local American Red Cross.

safety line—The safety line divides shallow water (5 feet [1.5 meters] or less) from deep water. It should be standard at all pools with deep water. If one is not available at your pool, you can make one using 1/4- to 1/2-inch (25 millimeters) nylon rope (one and a half times the length you need to extend across the pool) and small heavy plastic containers (fabric softener bottles) with lids. Tie the plastic containers individually on the rope, spaced about 2 feet (about half a meter) apart.

weighted objects—Weighted objects, such as rubberized rings and rubberized bricks, will sink to the bottom of the pool. They are most often used for object recovery. If budgets are a problem, you can make objects using old rubber car mats. Cut out shapes (numbers, letters, and the like) to enhance learning. Rubber bases and traffic cones (pylons) also sink to the bottom and are safe to use. They may be used to mark off a play area or design an obstacle course. Also check the gym storage. Many pieces of equipment used to mark spaces in the gymnasium can be used safely as pool equipment.

appendix b

Aquatic Equipment Supplies

The companies in this appendix have a number of options for purchasing equipment that is designed for water exercise or for pool play.

AquaMat
53 Barden Road
Barden Ridge 2234
NSW Australia
Phone: 612 9543 0995
Fax: 02 9543 0995
www.aquamat.com/aquamat.
  html
aquamat@ozemail.com.au

FlagHouse, Inc.
601 FlagHouse Drive
Hasbrouck Heights, NJ 07604-
  3116
800-793-7900, 201-288-7600
Fax: 800-793-7922
www.flaghouse.com
sales@flaghouse.com

Jay Fowler, The-SoundMan
7110 N. Brooklyn Avenue
Gladstone, MO 64118-2884
816-453-7110
Fax: 816-453-8686
jay@the-soundman.com

Adolph Kiefer and Associates
1700 Kiefer Drive
Zion, IL 60099
800-323-4071, 847-872-8866
Fax: 847-746-8888
www.kiefer.com
esales@kiefer.com

Sprint Aquatics
Sprint Rothhammer
P.O. Box 3840
San Luis Obispo, CA 93403-
  3840
800-235-2156, 805-541-5330
Fax: 805-541-5339
www.sprintaquatics.com
info@sprintaquatics.com

SPRI Products
1600 Northwind Boulevard
Libertyville, IL 60048
800-222-7774
www.spriproducts.com
teamspri@spriproducts.com

Associations Serving Aquatic Safety and Aquatic Exercise

The resources in this appendix provide educational training in fitness or water exercise and aquatic safety such as pool operations and lifeguarding.

American Alliance for Health, Physical Education, Recreation and Dance
(AAHPERD) Aquatic Council of AALF
1900 Association Drive
Reston, VA 20191-1598
800-213-7193
Fax: 703-476-9257
www.aahperd.org
info@aahperd.org

American Council on Exercise (ACE)
4851 Paramount Drive
San Diego, CA 92123
858-279-8227, 800-825-3636
Fax: 858-279-8064
www.acefitness.org
support@acefitness.org

American Red Cross National Headquarters
2025 E Street, NW
Washington, DC 20006
Phone: 202-303-4498
www.redcross.org
info@usa.redcross.org

Aquatic Exercise Association
P.O. Box 1609
Nokomis, FL 34274-1609
941-486-8600
888-AEA-WAVE
Fax: 941-486-8820
www.aeawave.com
info@aeawave.com

National Intramural-Recreational Sports Association (NIRSA)

4185 SW Research Way
Corvallis, OR 97333-1067
541-766-8211
Fax: 541-766-8284
www.nirsa.org
nirsa@nirsa.org

National Recreation and Park Association

22377 Belmont Ridge Road
Ashburn, VA 20148
703-858-0784
Fax: 703-858-0794
www.nrpa.org
info@nrpa.org

National Swimming Pool Foundation

4775 Granby Circle
Colorado Springs, CO 80919-3131
719-540-9119
Fax: 719-540-2787
www.nspf.com
media@nspf.org

United States Water Fitness Association

P.O. Box 243279
Boynton Beach, FL 33424-3279
561-732-9908
Fax: 561-732-0950
www.uswfa.com
info@uswfa.org

YMCA of the USA

101 N. Wacker Drive
Chicago, IL 60606
800-872-9622
Fax: 312-977-9063
www.ymca.net
fulfillment@ymca.net

appendix d

Skills Assessment Grid

Rate each person using the following scale:

+ Good

/ Acceptable

−Needs improvement

Individuals who can perform all skills with a + are ready for deep-water games and stunts.

Skills	PARTICIPANT NAMES						
Jump-in entry, chest-deep water							
Air exchange, mouth and nose							
Breath holding 5 seconds or longer							
Float unsup-ported on front							
Float unsup-ported on back							
Swim front crawl 25 yards or more							
Swim back-stroke 25 yards or more							

(continued)

	PARTICIPANT NAMES						
Skills							
Roll from front to back while swimming							
Jump into deep water, level off, and swim							
Swim under-water for 3 or more body lengths							
Tread water for more than 1 minute							
Change direc-tion while swimming on front							

From T. Lees, 2007, *Water fun* (Champaign, IL: Human Kinetics).

about the author

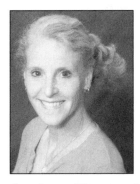

Terri Lees has been teaching aquatic activities and coaching swimming for more than 30 years. She taught and coached high school swimming for 12 years and spent 13 years at Wichita State University as the aquatic coordinator for campus recreation, where she taught and created aquatic programs for students and instructors.

Lees has been a contributor to the American Red Cross Water Safety Instructor and Swimming and Diving texts and served as an on-camera host for the Aqua Fitness video. She is currently the chair-elect for the Council for Aquatic Professionals of AAHPERD and has presented at numerous state, district, and national conventions. Lees also serves as the chair for the development committee of the aquatic fitness instructor credential. She is a master teacher of adapted aquatics and a master instructor of aquatic fitness for the AAHPERD Council for Aquatic Professionals.

Lees is the aquatic supervisor at North Kansas City Community Center in North Kansas City, Missouri. She is personally involved as a competitive swimmer and is coaching a 50+ age-group team at the community center. She has designed and created all of the water exercise programs for the center and provides personal training in the water for people with disabilities.

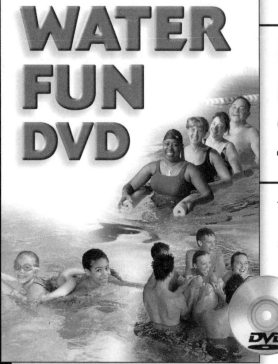
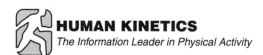